T0173469

Pharmaceutics – Drug Delivery and Targeting

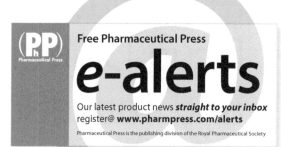

FASTtrack

Pharmaceutics – Drug Delivery and Targeting

Yvonne Perrie
Chair in Drug Delivery
Aston Pharmacy School
Aston University
Birmingham, UK

Thomas Rades
Chair in Pharmaceutical Sciences
The New Zealand National School of Pharmacy
University of Otago, Dunedin, New Zealand

Pharmaceutical Press

Published by Pharmaceutical Press

66-68 East Smithfield, London E1W 1AW, UK

(**PP**) is a trade mark of Pharmaceutical Press
Pharmaceutical Press is the publishing division of the Royal Pharmaceutical
Society

First edition published 2010
Second edition published 2012
Reprinted 2014

Typeset by Newgen Imaging Systems, India
Printed in Great Britain by TJ International, Padstow, Cornwall

ISBN 978 0 85711 059 6

Contents

Introduction to the *FASTtrack* series

FASTtrack is a new series of revision guides created for undergraduate pharmacy students. The books are intended to be used in conjunction with textbooks and reference books as an aid to revision to help guide students through their exams. They provide essential information required in each particular subject area. The books will also be useful for pre-registration trainees preparing for the General Pharmaceutical Council's (GPhC) registration examination, and to practising pharmacists as a quick reference text.

The content of each title focuses on what pharmacy students really need to know in order to pass exams. Features include*:
- concise bulleted information
- key points
- tips for the student
- multiple choice questions (MCQs) and worked examples
- case studies
- simple diagrams.

The titles in the *FASTtrack* series reflect the full spectrum of modules for the undergraduate pharmacy degree.

Titles include:
Applied Pharmaceutical Practice
Complementary and Alternative Medicine
Law and Ethics in Pharmacy Practice
Managing Symptoms in the Pharmacy
Pharmaceutical Compounding and Dispensing
Pharmaceutics: Dosage Form and Design
Pharmaceutics: Drug Delivery and Targeting
Pharmacology
Physical Pharmacy (based on Florence & Attwood's *Physicochemical Principles of Pharmacy*)
Therapeutics

There is also an accompanying website which includes extra MCQs, further title information and sample content: www.fasttrackpharmacy.com.

If you have any feedback regarding this series, please contact us at feedback@fasttrackpharmacy.com.

*Note: not all features are in every title in the series.

Preface

The best drugs can't exert their beneficial effects if they are not reaching their target site in the body at an appropriate concentration and for a sufficient length of time. It is clear that if a tablet is still in the package it is of no benefit for the patient. Less obvious is that this may also be the case after the tablet has been swallowed.

In the stomach the tablet might not disintegrate and the drug might not be released from the dosage form. Or the drug simply has too low aqueous solubility in the gastrointestinal fluids. If the drug is not in solution it will (generally) not be able to overcome the epithelial membranes of the gastrointestinal tract and it cannot enter into the body and reach the target site of its activity. *How can we improve the solubility of poorly water-soluble drugs?*

Some drugs chemically or enzymatically degrade in the stomach. Others lead to gastric irritation. *How can these drugs still be administered via the oral route?*

In other cases the drug may dissolve very fast and is absorbed very quickly from the gastrointestinal tract. Whilst this seems a good thing (and indeed it often is), it can lead to high plasma concentration peaks of the drug followed by fast elimination of the drug, and consequently a short duration of action. So the patient has to take the drug very frequently and there will be strong fluctuations in the plasma concentration of the drug over time. *Can we formulate a dosage form to improve this situation?*

Some drugs cannot be delivered by the oral route as they are metabolised in the liver, before reaching the systemic circulation. *What can be done?*

Again other drugs may have a strong side-effect profile, which may prohibit efficient treatment. *Can we improve this situation, and direct the drug to its target site, rather than having it distributed evenly throughout the body?*

This book tries to answer these and other questions in a concise and structured way. We will systematically review important concepts and facts relating to the delivery and targeting of drugs. The emphasis of this book has not been placed on the anatomical routes of delivery, but instead on the principles of drug release and targeting, namely: immediate release, delayed release, sustained release, controlled release and targeted release. Because of its overwhelming importance in drug delivery today, we have placed some focus on oral delivery (for immediate release, delayed release, sustained release), but other routes of delivery will also be covered where appropriate (for controlled and targeted release). Relevant examples of delivery systems will be given throughout the book with a focus on delivery systems that have actually reached clinical reality.

This book aims to highlight differences and principles in a concise way (including some mind maps at the end of the book), and so we have to apologise to the experts in the field if we have drawn boundaries for clarity where a grey zone is more appropriate. However, in the words of Picasso, we feel that students should know the boundaries before they can (and should) cross them.

In this second edition, we have had the opportunity to add a few additional examples to demonstrate further the application of drug delivery and targeting in clinical practice, and we gratefully acknowledge Mr Korbinian Löbmann and Mr Nicky Thomas (University of Otago) for their help with undertaking this review.

Yvonne Perrie
Thomas Rades

About the authors

Professor YVONNE PERRIE is the Chair in Drug Delivery within Aston Pharmacy School, Aston University, Birmingham, UK. She has a BSc (first-class honours) in Pharmacy (1994) from Strathclyde University, Scotland and registered with the Royal Pharmaceutical Society of Great Britain in 1995.

In 1998 Yvonne received her PhD from the University of London, UK where she investigated the use of liposomes for gene delivery under the supervision of Professor Gregory Gregoriadis. After working for a newly established drug delivery company, Lipoxen, Yvonne joined Aston University as a lecturer in 2000 and since 2007 holds the Chair in Drug Delivery.

Yvonne is currently the Head of Pharmacy within Aston University and was previously awarded the Aston University Teaching Excellence Award.

Yvonne's research is focused on the development of particulate carrier systems to facilitate the delivery of drugs and vaccines and aims to provide practical solutions to current healthcare problems. Yvonne is also Editor in Chief of the *Journal of Liposome Research*.

Professor THOMAS RADES is the Chair in Pharmaceutical Sciences at the National School of Pharmacy, University of Otago, New Zealand. He has a BSc in Pharmacy from the University of Hamburg, Germany and is a registered pharmacist.

In 1994 Thomas received a PhD from the University of Braunschweig, Germany for his work on thermotropic and lyotropic liquid crystalline drugs. After working as a research scientist in Preclinical Development and Formulation at F. Hoffmann-La Roche in Basel, Switzerland, he became Senior Lecturer in Pharmaceutical Sciences at Otago in 1999 and since 2003 holds the Chair in Pharmaceutical Sciences.

For his undergraduate and postgraduate teaching in pharmaceutics he was awarded the University of Otago Teaching Excellence Award and the New Zealand Tertiary Teaching Excellence Award for Sustained Excellence.

Thomas has developed an international reputation for his research in drug delivery and physical characterisation of drugs. He has currently published more than 200 papers in international peer review journals. His research interests include nanoparticles as delivery systems for drugs and vaccines, and the solid state of drugs and dosage forms.

chapter 1

Controlling drug delivery

Overview

In this chapter we will:
- differentiate drug delivery systems according to their physical state
- differentiate drug delivery systems according to their route of administration
- differentiate drug delivery systems according to their type of drug release
- discuss drug transport across epithelial barriers.

Introduction

Pharmacotherapy can be defined as the treatment and prevention of illness and disease by means of drugs of chemical or biological origin.

It ranks among the most important methods of medical treatment, together with surgery, physical treatment, radiation and psychotherapy. There are many success stories concerning the use of drugs and vaccines in the treatment, prevention and in some cases even eradication of diseases (e.g. smallpox, which is currently the only human infectious disease completely eradicated). Although it is almost impossible to estimate the exact extent of the impact of pharmacotherapy on human health, there can be no doubt that pharmacotherapy, together with improved sanitation, better diet and better housing, has improved people's health, life expectancy and quality of life.

Unprecedented developments in genomics and molecular biology today offer a plethora of new drug targets. The use of modern chemical synthetic methods (such as combinatorial chemistry) enables the syntheses of a large number of new drug candidates in shorter times than ever before. At the same time, a better understanding of the immune system and rapid progress in molecular biology, cell

KeyPoints

- Continued developments in chemistry, molecular biology and genomics support the discovery and developments of new drugs and new drug targets.
- The drug delivery system employed can control the pharmacological action of a drug, influencing its pharmacokinetic and subsequent therapeutic profile.

Tip

Combinatorial chemistry is a way to build a variety of structurally related drug compounds rapidly and systematically. These are assembled from a range of molecular entities which are put together in different combinations. A 'library' of compounds of tens of thousands of different molecules is then screened to identify compounds that bind to therapeutic targets.

biology and microbiology allow the development of modern vaccines against old and new challenges.

However, for all these exciting new drug and vaccine candidates, it is necessary to develop suitable dosage forms or drug delivery systems to allow the effective, safe and reliable application of these bioactive compounds to the patient. It is important to realise that the active ingredient (regardless of whether this is a small-molecular-weight 'classical' drug or a modern 'biopharmaceutical' drug like a therapeutic peptide, protein or antigen) is just one part of the medicine administered to the patient and it is the formulation of the drug into a dosage form or drug delivery system that translates drug discovery and pharmacological research into clinical practice.

Indeed the drug delivery system employed plays a vital role in controlling the pharmacological effect of the drug as it can influence the pharmacokinetic profile of the drug, the rate of drug release, the site and duration of drug action and subsequently the side-effect profile. An optimal drug delivery system ensures that the active drug is available at the site of action for the correct time and duration. The drug concentration at the appropriate site should be above the minimal effective concentration (MEC) and below the minimal toxic concentration (MTC). This concentration interval is known as the therapeutic range and the concept is illustrated in Figure 1.1, showing the drug

Tip

Usually the drug concentration in the body is determined in the plasma. This is done as the plasma is comparatively easy to access and drug concentrations can be reliably measured using techniques such as high-performance liquid chromatography (HPLC). However, the desired site of action for most drugs is not the plasma and in principle it would be better to determine the drug concentration at the site of action of the drug.

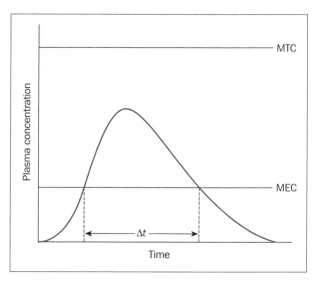

Figure 1.1 Drug plasma levels after oral administration of a drug form an immediate-release dosage form. The therapeutic range is the concentration interval between the minimal effective concentration (MEC) and the minimal toxic concentration (MTC). Δt is the time interval the drug is in the therapeutic range.

plasma levels after oral administration of a drug from an immediate-release dosage form.

Achieving the desired concentration of a drug is dependent on the frequency of dosing, the drug clearance rates, the route of administration and the drug delivery system employed. Within this book the terms drug delivery system, dosage form and medicine are used interchangeably. However the term dosage form is often used to refer to the physical appearance of the medicine whereas the term delivery system is often used to refer to the way the medicine releases the drug and delivers it to the body or more specifically to the target organ, tissue, cell or even cellular organelle.

Differentiating delivery systems according to their physical state

For dosage forms it is common to differentiate the various types by classifying them according to their physical state into gaseous (e.g. anaesthetics), liquid (e.g. solutions, emulsions, suspensions), semisolid (e.g. creams, ointments, gels and pastes) and solid dosage forms (e.g. powders, granules, tablets and capsules). Most dosage forms contain several phases.

Sometimes the phases of a dosage form are of the same state, for example for an emulsion which contains two liquid phases (oil and water). Whilst both phases are liquid, they differ in their physical properties, for example density and electrical conductivity, and are separated from each other by an interface. However, more often the dosage form contains phases of different states. For example, a suspension contains a liquid and a solid phase. Therefore classification into gaseous, liquid, semisolid or solid dosage forms may sometimes appear somewhat arbitrary. Finally, in these multiphase dosage forms usually one or more phases are dispersed, whilst other phases are continuous. In a suspension the solid phase is dispersed and the liquid phase is continuous, and in an oil-in-water emulsion the oil phase is dispersed and the water phase is continuous. In some dosage forms the determination of the type and number of phases is not as straightforward.

KeyPoints

- Dosage forms can be classified according to their physical state.
- Most dosage forms contain several phases.
- Systems containing a dispersed phase will give rise to physical instability issues.
- All systems move to a state of minimum free energy.

Tip

A phase is a volume element of a system (here the dosage form), separated from other volume elements of the system by a phase boundary (interface to another phase). The physical properties within the phase do not vary, which means that the phase is physically homogeneous. From the requirement of homogeneity within a phase it follows that the number of molecules within the phase is large compared to the number of molecules forming the interface between the phases and surrounding other phases.

Tip

To understand dosage forms from a physical perspective, try to identify the number of phases in a dosage form, their state and if they are dispersed or continuous.

Tips

Here are some examples of how dosage forms in their simplest terms can be differentiated according to the state and dispersion of their phases:

■ A drug solution is a one-phase system as the dissolved drug does not fulfil the requirements for a phase. In a solution the molecularly dispersed drug will not separate out to form larger particles if the concentration of the drug is not changed (e.g. by evaporation of the solvent) and the environmental conditions (e.g. temperature) are constant.

■ A suspension is a two-phase system containing a continuous liquid phase and a dispersed solid phase.

■ An emulsion is a two-phase system containing two liquid phases, one dispersed and one continuous.

■ Ointments are generally two-phase or multiphase gels, with at least two continuous phases (usually a crystalline or liquid crystalline surfactant phase and a lipid phase).

■ Creams additionally contain a water phase which may be dispersed (water-in-oil cream) or continuous (oil-in-water cream).

■ Tablets are essentially compressed powers, and might thus be classified as containing a solid and gaseous continuous phase. Of course a tablet contains several solid phases, as drug particles are usually present together with other solid phases (e.g. filler, binder, disintegrant, glidant and lubricant particles).

For example, the phases of creams can be difficult to determine, with the presence of a dispersed water (or oil) phase in addition to several continuous phases (oil, water and surfactant phases). For liposomal dispersions, the state of the phospholipids used to form the liposomes will determine if a liposomal dispersion is a suspension (if the lipids are in a crystalline state) or an emulsion (if the lipids are in a fluid, liquid crystalline state).

It is important to note that the presence of a dispersed phase will lead to physical instability in the system. For example, in an oil-in-water emulsion, the dispersed oil droplets have a larger interfacial area to the water than if the droplets had coalesced into one large continuous phase. This increased interfacial area leads to an increased interfacial free energy, according to the relationship:

$$G_i = A\gamma$$

where G_i is the interfacial free energy of the system, A is the interfacial area between the dispersed phase (here the oil droplets) and the continuous phase (here the water phase) and γ is the interfacial tension between the two phases. The interfacial free energy of the system (here the emulsion) can be minimised by coalescence of the droplets into larger droplets and finally into one continuous oil phase, as this maximally reduces the total interfacial area. This is of course undesirable from a formulation viewpoint. Coalescence of droplets in an emulsion is a pharmaceutical instability, but from a thermodynamic viewpoint the system has been stabilised, as the interfacial free energy has been reduced. In practical terms an emulsion is pharmaceutically stabilised by adding emulsifiers to the systems, that either lower the interfacial tension (note: if γ gets smaller, G_i will get smaller), or that act as a physical barrier against coalescence. In either case, increasing the interfacial area will still increase the surface free energy.

Differentiating delivery systems according to their route of administration

Another way of differentiating dosage forms is according to their site or route of administration. Drugs can be administered directly into the body, through injection or infusion. This form of drug administration is termed parenteral drug delivery. Depending on the site of administration into the body one can differentiate between intravenous, intramuscular, subcutaneous, intradermal and intraperitoneal administration. Usually aqueous solutions are used for intravenous delivery, but it is also possible that the dosage form contains a dispersed phase (solid or liquid), provided the dispersed particles are small enough (e.g. smaller than 100–150 nm) to avoid embolism. For other routes of parenteral administration the delivery systems can be aqueous or oily or even solid (the latter dosage forms are termed implants).

Drugs can also be administered on to the skin to enter into the body. Mostly semisolid dosage forms are used for this, including creams, ointments, gels and pastes. However, liquid dosage forms, such as emulsions, or solid dosage forms, such as transdermal controlled drug delivery systems (patches), can also be used. These will be discussed in more depth in Chapter 6. It has to be taken into account, though, that one of the main functions of the skin as an organ is to prevent particles or compounds entering the body, rather than allowing them to be absorbed into the body. The stratum corneum of the skin forms a formidable barrier against uptake and thus transdermal delivery is difficult to achieve. Penetration enhancers often have to be added to the delivery system to improve delivery into or through the skin. In transdermal controlled drug delivery systems ideally the dosage form controls the uptake into the skin (rather than the uptake being controlled by the stratum corneum).

The most important route of drug administration into the body is through mucosal membranes. Mucosal membranes are much less of a barrier to uptake than the skin and some mucosal membranes (such as the ones in the small intestine) are indeed specialised sites for absorption. There are many mucosal membranes that can be used for drug administration. Of the highest importance are the mucosal membranes of the gastrointestinal tract, allowing oral drug delivery. The suitability and convenience of this route of delivery make oral dosage forms the most common of all drug delivery systems. Also the buccal, sublingual, rectal and vaginal mucosa and indeed the lung and nasal mucosal membranes can act as absorption sites. For all of these mucosal membranes dosage forms have been developed, such as buccal and sublingual tablets, suppositories, vaginal rings, inhalers and nasal sprays, to name a few.

If drug delivery systems are designed to give a local drug effect and not systemic activity, they can be described as topical delivery systems. This is the case for many dermal dosage forms.

Oral drug delivery

As stated above, the oral route is the most popular route to administer drugs. However, some factors should be considered when looking to administer drugs via this route. In particular the transit time in the gastrointestinal tract may vary considerably:

- between patients and within the same patient, with the gastric residence time being the most variable
- with the state of the dosage form (liquid dosage forms are emptied out of the stomach faster than solid dosage forms)
- with the fasted or fed state of the patient.

The pH conditions in the gastrointestinal tract also vary considerably, from a low pH in the stomach (1.5–2 in the fasted state to around 5 in the fed state) to a higher pH in the small and large intestine. The pH in the small intestine varies from 4 to 7, with an average value of approximately 6.5. This may affect stability and will influence the degree of ionisation of ionisable drugs which in turn will influence their absorption (unionised forms of drugs are usually taken up better than ionised forms of the same drug) and solubility (unionised forms are usually less soluble than ionised forms of the same drug).

First-pass metabolism

Importantly, drugs that are taken up into the body through the gastrointestinal mucosa will be transported to the liver via the portal vein before going into general circulation. As the liver is the main metabolic organ of the body, if the drug is susceptible to metabolic degradation in the liver, this may considerably reduce the activity of the drug. This phenomenon is known as the hepatic first-pass effect. The rectal route may also show varying degrees of the first-pass effect, while for other routes of administration (intravenous, vaginal, nasal, buccal and sublingual) the drug is distributed in the body before reaching the liver, and therefore for certain drugs these may be the preferred route of administration. However, whilst the liver is the main metabolic organ of the body, metabolism may also take place in the gastrointestinal lumen and indeed in the mucosal membranes.

Differentiating drug delivery systems according to their mechanism of drug release

Another systematic that can be used to differentiate drug delivery systems is according to the way the drug is released. Broadly, one can differentiate as follows:

- Immediate release – drug is released immediately after administration.
- Modified release – drug release only occurs some time after the administration or for a prolonged period of time or to a specific target in the body. Modified-release systems can be further classified as:
- Delayed release: drug is released only at some point after the initial administration.
- Extended release: prolongs the release to reduce dosing frequency.

These terms are also used by the pharmacopoeias and the FDA. Whilst immediate-release dosage forms are designed to give a fast onset of drug action, modifications in drug release are often desirable to increase the stability, safety and efficacy of the drug, to improve the therapeutic outcome of the drug treatment and/or to increase patient compliance and convenience of administration.

Tip

After oral administration first-pass metabolism may occur in the liver and the gut. For example, glyceryl trinitrate is predominantly metabolised in the liver and is therefore often formulated for sublingual delivery. In contrast, benzylpenicillin and insulin are primarily metabolised in the gut lumen while orlistat is metabolised within the gastrointestinal mucosal membrane.

KeyPoints

- Dosage forms can control the rate of release of a drug and/ or the location of release.
- They can be classified into immediate-release and modified-release dosage forms.
- The modified-release systems can be further divided into delayed-, extended- and targeted-release systems.
- Extended-release systems can be further divided into sustained- and controlled-release systems.
- Modifications in drug release profiles can be used to improve the stability, safety, efficacy and therapeutic profile of a drug.

Tips

The various forms of release as defined by the FDA

Immediate release
Allows the drug to dissolve in the gastrointestinal contents, with no intention of delaying or prolonging the dissolution or absorption of the drug.

Modified release

Dosage forms whose drug release characteristics of time course and/or location are chosen to accomplish therapeutic or convenience objectives not offered by conventional dosage forms such as a solution or an immediate-release dosage form. Modified-release solid oral dosage forms include both delayed- and extended-release drug products.

Delayed release

Release of a drug (or drugs) at a time other than immediately following oral administration.

Extended release

Extended-release products are formulated to make the drug available over an extended period after ingestion. This allows a reduction in dosing frequency compared to a drug presented as a conventional dosage form (e.g. as a solution or an immediate-release dosage form).

No definition for controlled release or targeted release is provided by the FDA or pharmacopoeias.

KeyPoints

- Immediate-release delivery systems give a fast onset of action.
- For a therapeutic action the drug should be in solution, therefore disintegration of the dosage form and dissolution of the drug may have to occur first depending on the dosage form.
- Immediate-release systems usually release the drug in a single action following a first-order kinetics profile.
- The time of action of the drug is limited to the time that the concentration of the drug is above the MEC.

Immediate release

Many dosage forms are designed to release the drug immediately or at least as quickly as possible after administration. This is useful if a fast onset of action is required for therapeutic reasons. For example, a tablet containing a painkiller should disintegrate quickly in the gastrointestinal tract to allow a fast uptake into the body.

The onset of action is very fast for intravenous injections and infusions and the pharmacological effect may be seen in a matter of seconds after administration. The reasons for this are twofold:

1. The drug is already in solution, so strictly speaking the drug does not have to be released from the dosage form at all.
2. The drug is directly administered into the body, so no time is lost due to drug permeation through the skin or mucosal membranes, before the target organs can be reached.

In oral solutions the drug is also already released and the solution will simply mix with the gastrointestinal fluids. However, powders and granules need to dissolve first before the drug is released by dissolution. For tablets it is initially necessary that the tablet disintegrates (if it is formed from compressed granules this will initially happen to the level of the granules, from which further disintegration into powder particles and finally drug dissolution occurs). For capsules to release their drug content it is necessary for the capsule shell material (for example, gelatin or hydroxypropylmethylcellulose (HPMC)) first to disintegrate. Thereafter the drug can either dissolve from the usually solid powders or granules in the case of hard gelatin or HPMC capsules or it can be dispersed from the usually liquid, lipophilic content of a soft gelatin capsule. These types of immediate-release dosage forms have an onset of action in the order of minutes to hours.

Immediate-release dosage forms usually release (dissolve or disperse) the drug in a single action following a first-order kinetics profile. This means the drug is released initially very quickly and then passes through the mucosal membrane into the body, reaching the highest plasma level (termed C_{max}) in a comparatively short time (termed t_{max}). Uptake through the mucosal membranes may be due to passive diffusion or by receptor-mediated active transport mechanisms (see section on modified release). Once taken up into the body the drug is distributed throughout the body and elimination of the drug by metabolism and excretion occurs. The elimination process also usually follows first-order kinetics. Therefore the plasma levels measured over time after administration of an immediate-release dosage form (the plasma concentration time curve) basically are the sum of a first-order absorption and a first-order elimination process. The resulting function is known as the Bateman function. Figure 1.2 shows an idealised plasma concentration versus time profile of an immediate-release oral dosage form.

An important consideration for immediate-release dosage forms is that the time of action of the drug is limited to the time that the concentration of the drug is above the MEC. If the drug has a short biological half-life, this time interval may be short, requiring

Tips

First-order kinetics
The rate of the process is proportional to the concentration of one of the reactants, in our case the drug.

Bateman function
This function was initially used to describe the concentration of a radioactive material B that stems from a first-order decay of another radioactive material A and that in its own right further decays to another material C. If both decay processes ($A \rightarrow B$ and $B \rightarrow C$) follow first-order kinetics, exactly the same function results as for the plasma concentration time curve of a drug from an immediate-release oral dosage form. The $A \rightarrow B$ decay is equivalent to the absorption process and the $B \rightarrow C$ process is equivalent to the elimination process.

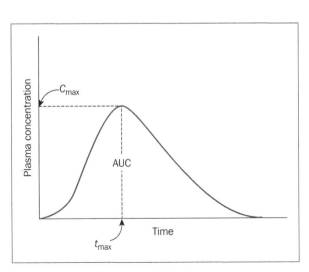

Figure 1.2 Idealised plasma concentration versus time profile of an immediate-release oral dosage form. The highest drug plasma concentration is termed C_{max}. The time at which C_{max} is reached is termed t_{max}. The area under the plasma concentration versus time profile is termed AUC and reflects the total amount of drug absorbed.

frequent dosing and potentially leading to low patient compliance and suboptimal therapeutic outcome.

The biological half-life of a drug is defined as the time required to reduce the plasma concentration by 50% by metabolism or excretion. Many studies show that a large proportion of patients do not take drugs as directed (for example three times a day), especially if the disease is (at least initially) not accompanied by strong symptoms, for example in the treatment of high blood pressure or glaucoma. To reduce the frequency of drug administration it is often not possible simply to increase the dose of an immediate-release dosage form as the peak plasma concentrations may be too high and lead to unacceptable side-effects. Therefore the drug concentration within the plasma should be above the MEC and below the MTC, i.e. within the therapeutic range (Figure 1.1).

KeyPoints

- Modified-release systems are designed to influence the release profile of a drug from its delivery system.
- Oral delayed-release systems can delay release until specific regions of the gastrointestinal tract are reached.
- Extended release of a drug can be achieved using sustained- or controlled-release drug delivery systems.
- Controlled-release systems aim to control the plasma concentration of the drug after administration by various possible routes.

Tip

Immediate-release oral delivery systems can also have polymer coatings. In this case the polymer may be used to mask an unpleasant taste or odour, to facilitate swallowing of the drug or to improve identification of the medicine. These coats dissolve quickly in the stomach and do not delay the release of the drug.

Modified release

Dosage forms can be designed to modify the release of the drug over a given time or after the dosage form reaches the required location.

Delayed release

Delayed-release dosage forms can be defined as systems which are formulated to release the active ingredient at a time other than immediately after administration. Delayed release from oral dosage forms can control where the drug is released, e.g. when the dosage form reaches the small intestine (enteric-coated dosage forms) or the colon (colon-specific dosage forms).

Delayed-release systems can be used to protect the drug from degradation in the low pH environment of the stomach or to protect the stomach from irritation by the drug. In these cases drug release should be delayed until the dosage form has reached the small intestine. Often polymers are used to achieve this aim. The dosage form (for example, a tablet or the granules before tableting) can be coated with a suitable polymer. The polymer dissolves as a function of pH, so when the dosage forms travel from the low-pH environment of the stomach to the higher-pH environment of the small intestine, the polymer coat dissolves and the drug can be released. Once this occurs, the release is again immediate and the resulting plasma concentration versus time curve is similar to the one for immediate-release dosage forms.

The development of colon-specific drugs and dosage forms may be advantageous for the treatment of local and systemic diseases, including colorectal cancer and Crohn's disease. Especially for peptide and protein drugs, this form of release may also be advantageous for systemic administration given the more favourable pH conditions in the colon compared to the stomach and the generally lower enzymatic activity compared to the small intestine.

Figure 1.3 shows an idealised plasma concentration versus time profile of a delayed-release oral dosage form. T_{max} (but not C_{max}) is strongly dependent on the gastric emptying times which, as stated above, may be quite variable.

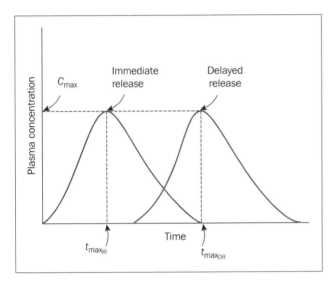

Figure 1.3 Idealised plasma concentration versus time profile of a delayed-release oral dosage form compared to an immediate-release dosage form. T_{maxIR} is the time for maximum plasma concentration of the drug released from an immediate-release dosage form and T_{maxDR} is the time for maximum plasma concentration of the drug released from a delayed-release dosage form.

Extended release

Extended-release systems allow for the drug to be released over prolonged time periods. By extending the release profile of a drug, the frequency of dosing can be reduced. For immediate-release dosage forms the time interval the plasma concentration is in the therapeutic range of the drug can be quite short. Therefore frequent dosing, with its associated compliance problems, is required. This is especially an issue in chronic diseases when patients need to take the medicine for prolonged periods of time, often for the rest of their life. Extended release can be achieved using sustained- or controlled-release dosage forms.

Sustained release

These systems maintain the rate of drug release over a sustained period (Figure 1.4). For example, if the release of the drug from the dosage form is sustained such that the release takes place throughout the entire gastrointestinal tract, one could reduce C and prolong the time interval of drug concentration in the therapeutic range. This in turn may reduce the frequency of dosing, for example from three times a day to once a day. Sustained-release dosage forms achieve this mostly by the use of suitable polymers, which are used either to coat granules or tablets (reservoir systems) or to form a matrix in which the drug is dissolved or dispersed (matrix systems). The release kinetics of the drug from these systems may differ:

- Reservoir systems often follow a zero-order kinetics (linear release as a function of time).
- Matrix systems often follow a linear release as a function of the square root of time.

Figure 1.4 Idealised plasma concentration versus time profile of a sustained-release oral dosage form compared to an immediate-release dosage form.

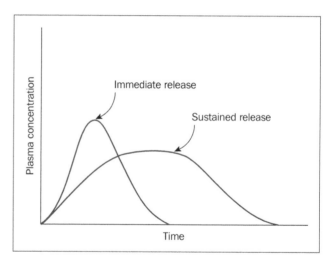

Controlled release

Controlled-release systems also offer a sustained-release profile but, in contrast to sustained-release forms, controlled-release systems are designed to lead to predictably constant plasma concentrations, independently of the biological environment of the application site. This means that they are actually controlling the drug concentration in the body, not just the release of the drug from the dosage form, as is the case in a sustained-release system. Another difference between sustained- and controlled-release dosage forms is that the former are basically restricted to oral dosage forms whilst controlled-release systems are used in a variety of administration routes, including transdermal, oral and vaginal administration.

Controlled release of drugs from a dosage form may be achieved by the use of so-called therapeutic systems. These are drug delivery systems in which the drug is released in a predetermined pattern over a fixed period of time. The release kinetics is usually zero-order. In contrast to sustained-release systems, the dose in the therapeutic systems is of less importance than the release rate from the therapeutic system. Ideally the release rate from the dosage form should be the rate-determining step for the absorption of the drug and in fact for the drug concentration in the plasma and target site. However, controlled-release systems are not necessarily target-specific, which means that they do not 'exclusively' deliver the drug to the target organ. This may be achieved by so-called targeted delivery systems which aim to exploit the characteristics of the drug carrier and the drug target to control the biodistribution of the drug. Figure 1.5 shows an idealised plasma concentration versus time profile of a controlled-release dosage form.

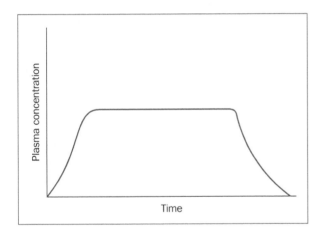

Figure 1.5 Idealised plasma concentration versus time profile of a controlled-release dosage form.

Optimum release profile

From immediate release and delayed release to sustained release and controlled release, we have seen that the resulting plasma concentration versus time curves have become increasingly flatter, prolonging the time the drug is in the therapeutic range after a single administration of the dosage form. This has led to the popular slogan: 'The flatter the better'. However, for some diseases it is advantageous to have varying release of the drug depending on the needs of the patient or circadian rhythms in the body. For example, insulin is needed in higher concentration after a meal and blood pressure has been found to be higher in the morning and afternoon and drops off during the night. Patients with rheumatoid arthritis suffer from pain more strongly in the morning than in the night, whilst the situation is reversed for patients with osteoarthritis. It has also long been known that cortisol levels are higher in the morning and decline throughout the day. This has led to research into so-called feedback-regulated drug delivery systems in which the drug concentration (ideally at the drug target site) is measured through a sensor and, depending on the ideal drug concentration, release is either increased or slowed down. It is also possible that instead of the actual drug concentration a therapeutic effect is measured that then acts as a feedback for the drug release. These systems, however, have not yet entered the market.

KeyPoints

- Controlling the release rate of a drug does not ensure that the drug reaches the target site or is retained there.
- Passively targeted drug delivery systems can utilise the natural distribution mechanisms within the body.
- Active targeting of delivery systems uses targeting groups such as antibodies and ligands to direct the system to the appropriate target.

Targeted-release dosage forms

Whilst controlling the rate of release of a drug from its delivery system can control plasma drug concentration levels, once released there is often little control over the distribution of the drug in the body. Very few drugs bind exclusively to the desired therapeutic target and this can give rise to reduced efficacy and increased toxicity.

Drug targeting aims to control the distribution of a drug within the body such that the majority of the dose selectively interacts with the target tissue at a cellular or subcellular level. By doing so, it is possible to enhance the activity and specificity of the drug and to reduce its toxicity and side-effects. Drug targeting can be achieved by designing systems that passively target sites by exploiting the natural conditions of the target organ or tissue to direct the drug to the target site. Alternatively drugs and certain delivery systems can be actively targeted using targeting groups such as antibodies to bind to specific receptors on cells.

The differentiation of dosage forms according to drug release places the emphasis on the delivery of the drug and will be followed in this book.

KeyPoints

- The epithelial lining presents a barrier to drug absorption.
- Epithelia are classified based on their shape, number of cells that form the epithelial barrier and their specialisation.
- Mucus secreted from goblet cells presents an additional barrier to drug absorption.

Drug absorption

By using the various drug delivery strategies outlined above, it is possible to influence the distribution of a delivery system and the release of a drug from its delivery system. However, we must also consider the process of drug absorption after the drug has been released. The absorption of drugs is dependent on the site of absorption and the nature of the drug. Nearly all internal and external body surfaces, and hence possible drug absorption routes, are lined with epithelial tissue. For example, drugs administered orally must cross the epithelium of the gastrointestinal tract before they can enter the systemic circulation.

Barriers to drug absorption

Epithelia are tissues composed of one or more layers of cells. These layers are supported by a basement membrane which lies on top of the supporting connective tissue. The function of epithelial cells includes absorption, secretion and protection and is dependent on their location within the body. The epithelia are classified by their:

1. *Shape*
    a. Squamous – these cells have a flat (squashed) shape.
    b. Columnar – these are narrow, tall cells.
    c. Cuboidal – these cells have a cubic shape, intermediate between squamous and columnar.

2. *Stratification (number of cell layers)*
    a. Simple – single layer of cells, termed epithelium.
    b. Stratified – multiple layers.

3. *Specialisation – some epithelia will have a specialised function*
    a. Keratinised cells contain keratin protein to improve the strength of the barrier.
    b. Ciliated cells have apical membrane extensions that can increase the overall absorption area and rhythmically beat to move mucus.

Tips

Examples of epithelia include:
- Blood vessels: this epithelium lines the circulatory system and consists of a single layer of squamous cells.
- Oral: this epithelium consists of a single layer of columnar cells and lines the stomach and intestine. Cells of the small intestine have villi and microvilli to increase their surface area.
- Buccal: this epithelium consists of stratified squamous cells that may be keratinised.

Mucus

Many of the epithelial linings considered as absorption sites have a mucus layer coating. Mucus is synthesised and secreted by goblet cells which are a specialised type of columnar epithelial cells. Mucus is viscous in nature and is composed of highly glycosylated peptides known as mucins and inorganic salts in water. The main role of mucus is to protect and lubricate the epithelial lining. In the respiratory tract it supports mucociliary clearance, by trapping substances and removing them through the mucociliary escalator. In the gastrointestinal tract, mucus both protects the stomach from the acidic conditions therein and helps lubricate the passage of food.

However, in terms of drug delivery, mucus serves as a physical barrier to absorption. A substance must first diffuse across the mucus barrier before it can reach the epithelia and be absorbed. Therefore the viscosity and thickness of the mucus layer and

KeyPoints

- Drugs can cross epithelia by transcellular and paracellular mechanisms.
- The paracellular mechanism involves passive diffusion between cells.
- Transcellular diffusion involves movement through cells and may require energy.
- The route of transport is dependent on the physicochemical nature of the drug.

any interactions the drug and/or delivery system may have with the mucus must be considered.

Mechanisms of drug absorption

The combination of the epithelial membranes and (where present) the mucus restricts the absorption of substances, including drugs. However there are mechanisms of absorption across the epithelial cells which involve:

- transcellular transport through cells
- paracellular transport between cells.

These mechanisms are summarised in Figure 1.6.

Figure 1.6 Transport processes across epithelial barriers.

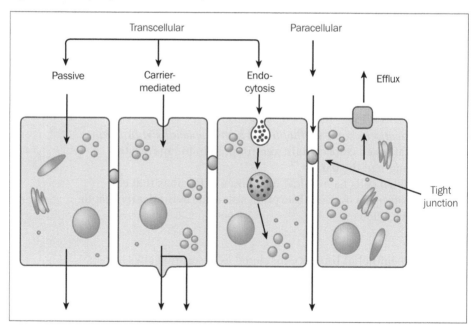

Transcellular route

Passive diffusion

This involves the diffusion of drugs across the lipid bilayer of the cell membrane and is driven by a concentration gradient with drugs moving from high to low concentration. The rate of diffusion is governed by Fick's law. Low-molecular-weight drugs are absorbed by passive diffusion and factors controlling the rate of diffusion include:

- drug concentration
- partition coefficient of the drug
- area of absorptive tissue.

In particular the lipophilicity of the drug is important since the drug must diffuse across the cell membrane and an optimum partition coefficient is usually observed for passive diffusion processes.

Carrier-mediated transport

This form of transport involves specific carrier proteins present in the cell membranes. Carrier-mediated transport can either act with a concentration gradient (facilitated diffusion) or against a concentration gradient (active absorption). For active absorption, as the transport is working against a concentration gradient, energy is required.

Any molecules, including drug molecules, which are similar to the natural substrate of the carrier protein are transported across the cell membrane. As this process involves a carrier protein, the mechanism is saturable at high concentrations and uptake via this route can be inhibited by competing substrates.

Endocytosis

This process involves internalisation of substances by engulfment by the cell membrane which forms membrane-based vesicles within the cell, known as endosomes. This allows larger molecules or particulates to enter the cell. There are several types of endocytosis:

- Receptor-mediated endocytosis: substances interact with specific surface receptors. As this involves receptors, the process is saturable. Drugs bind to receptors on the surface of the cell. This promotes invagination and vesicle formation in the cell. Within these vesicles, known as endosomes, the contents are subjected to low-pH conditions and digestive enzymes which can result in drug degradation/inactivation.

- Adsorptive endocytosis: this involves non-specific interactions with the cell surface receptors and therefore is non-saturable.
- Pinocytosis: this involves the uptake of solutes and single molecules. Large soluble macromolecules can be taken up by this process. This is a non-specific process that goes on continually in all cell types.
- Phagocytosis: with this process larger particulates may be taken up. Only specialised cells of the reticuloendothelial system (also known as the mononuclear phagocyte system) are capable of phagocytosis. This includes cells such as blood monocytes and macrophages.

Pore transport

Very small molecules may also be taken up through aqueous pores that are present in some cell membranes. These are ~0.4 nm in diameter so this transport mechanism is very restrictive. Only very small hydrophilic drugs can enter cells via this route.

Paracellular route

Drugs can also cross epithelia through gaps (known as gap junctions) between the cells. This route is governed by passive diffusion and small hydrophilic molecules can pass through these gap junctions. Transport across the epithelia can be enhanced using penetration enhancers which can damage the gap junctions; however possible toxicity implications should be considered with such methods.

Efflux

Substances can also be pushed back out of cells by an energy-dependent efflux system. There are various apical transmembrane proteins which can transport drugs out of the cell. Drugs that are subjected to efflux processes include cytotoxic drugs such as taxol, steroids, immunosuppressants and antibiotics.

Efflux is a major concern in the development of antimicrobial resistance. The genetic information for efflux pumps can be contained within chromosomes and/or plasmids. This allows for the efflux pump genes to be passed to various bacterial species. Expression of several efflux pumps in bacteria can lead to multidrug resistance.

KeyPoints

- The role of the drug delivery systems is to allow the effective, safe, and reliable application of the drug to the patient.
- To achieve this aim the drug must reach its target site.
- The system must be able to be produced in a technically feasible way and the quality of the formulation process must be assured.

Summary

No matter how dosage forms are classified, the role of the drug delivery systems is to allow the effective, safe, and reliable application of the drug to the patient.

For the development of dosage forms the formulation scientist needs to optimise the bioavailability of the drug. This means the delivery systems should allow and facilitate the drug to reach its target site in the body. For example, a tablet formulation containing an antihypertensive drug must disintegrate in the gastrointestinal tract, the drug needs to dissolve and the dissolved drug needs to permeate across the mucosal membrane of the gastrointestinal tract into the body.

Whilst some drugs are meant to act locally, e.g. in the oral cavity, in the gastrointestinal tract, in the eye or on the skin, nevertheless the prime role of the drug delivery system is to allow the drug to reach its target site.

Another role of the delivery systems is to allow the safe application of the drug. This includes that the drug in the formulation must be chemically, physically and microbiologically stable. Side-effects of the drug and drug interactions should be avoided or minimised by the use of suitable drug delivery systems. The delivery systems also need to improve the patient's compliance with the pharmacotherapy by the development of convenient applications. For example, one can improve patient compliance by developing an oral dosage form where previously only parenteral application was possible.

Finally, the delivery system needs to be reliable and its formulation needs to be technically feasible. This means the pharmaceutical quality of the delivery systems needs to be assured, drug release from the system needs to be reproducible and the influence of the body on drug release should be minimised (for example, food effects after oral administration). However, for any application of a drug delivery system on the market, the dosage form needs to be produced in large quantities and at low costs to make affordable medicines available. Therefore, it is also necessary to investigate the feasibility of the developed systems to be scaled up from the laboratory to the production scale. Figure 1.7 summarises the key attributes to be optimised to develop a drug into a medicine.

Tip

If a drug is in the gastrointestinal tract it is still outside the body.

Tip

Some confusion may arise from the use of the expression targeted drug delivery systems. In this book we define targeted delivery system as systems that allow selective targeting of the drug to a specific tissue, organ or specific cells inside the body to achieve a targeted drug *action*. If the *release* of the drug from the dosage form is targeted to a specific organ, these systems may be better called topical delivery systems (although some authors define only dermal application of dosage forms as being topical).

Figure 1.7 Key attributes that need to be optimised to develop a drug into a medicine.

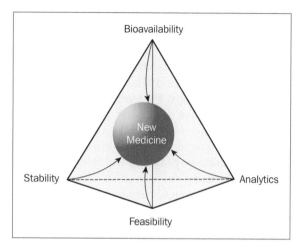

Self-assessment

After having read this chapter you should be able to:

- differentiate dosage forms according to their physical state and to give examples for each category
- differentiate dosage forms according to their route of administration and to list examples for each category
- differentiate dosage forms according to their drug release and to list examples for each category
- describe and explain plasma concentration versus time profiles of immediate-release oral dosage forms
- describe and explain plasma concentration versus time profiles of delayed-release oral dosage forms
- describe and explain plasma concentration versus time profiles of sustained-release oral dosage forms
- describe and explain plasma concentration versus time profiles of controlled-release oral dosage forms
- discuss the therapeutic range of a drug and how it is linked to the plasma concentration versus time profiles of oral dosage forms
- compare and contrast targeted and non-targeted drug release
- identify the essential features of transcellular and paracellular absorption via:
  - passive diffusion
  - carrier-mediated transport
  - endocytosis
  - paracellular absorption
  - efflux
- discuss the key attributes to be optimised to develop a drug into a medicine.

Questions

1. **Indicate which one of the following statements is not correct:**
a. The drug delivery system can play a vital role in controlling the pharmacological effect of the drug.
b. The drug delivery system can influence the pharmacokinetic profile of the drug, the rate of drug release, the site and duration of drug action and subsequently the side-effect profile.
c. An optimal drug delivery system ensures that the active drug is available at the site of action for the correct time and duration.
d. The drug concentration at the appropriate site should be below the minimal effective concentration (MEC).
e. The concentration interval between the MEC and the minimal toxic concentration (MTC) is known as the therapeutic range.

2. **Indicate which one of the following statements is not correct:**
a. A simple emulsion contains two liquid phases (oil and water).
b. In a water-in-oil emulsion, the oil phase is dispersed and the water phase is continuous.
c. A simple suspension contains a liquid and a solid phase.
d. In a suspension the solid phase is dispersed and the liquid phase is continuous.
e. In most multiphase dosage forms one or more phases are dispersed, whilst other phases are continuous.

3. **Indicate which one of the following statements is not correct:**
a. Dispersing one phase into the other will lead to a larger interfacial area between the two phases.
b. A larger interfacial area between the two phases leads to an increased interfacial free energy, according to the relationship: $G_i = A\gamma$.
c. In the equation $G_i = A\gamma$, G_i is the interfacial free energy of the system.
d. In the equation $G_i = A\gamma$, A is the interfacial area between the dispersed phase and the continuous phase.
e. In the equation $G_i = A\gamma$, γ is the surface tension of the continuous phase.

4. **Indicate which one of the following statements is not correct:**
a. The most important route of drug administration into the body is through mucosal membranes.
b. Mucosal membranes are a stronger barrier to drug uptake than the skin.
c. The mucosal membranes of the small intestine are specialised sites for absorption.

d. There are many mucosal membranes that can be used for drug administration.

e. Absorption of drugs through the mucosal membranes of the gastrointestinal tract allows for oral drug delivery.

5. **Indicate which one of the following statements is not correct:**

a. Drugs that are taken up into the body through the gastrointestinal mucosa will be transported to the liver via the portal vein before going into general circulation.

b. If the drug is susceptible to metabolic degradation in the liver, this may considerably enhance the activity of the drug. This phenomenon is known as the hepatic first-pass effect.

c. The rectal route may also show varying degrees of the first-pass effect.

d. In other routes of administration (intravenous, vaginal, nasal, buccal and sublingual) the drug is distributed in the body before reaching the liver.

e. Whilst the liver is the main metabolic organ of the body, metabolism may also take place in the gastrointestinal lumen and indeed in the mucosal membranes.

6. **Indicate which one of the following statements is not correct:**

a. Many dosage forms are designed to release the drug immediately after administration. This is useful if a fast onset of action is required for therapeutic reasons.

b. The onset of action is very fast for intravenous injections and infusions and a pharmacological effect may be seen in a matter of seconds after administration.

c. The onset of action is fast for oral delivery of immediate-release dosage forms, such as simple tablets, and a pharmacological effect may be seen in a matter of minutes to hours.

d. If the drug has a long biological half-life, the time interval between administrations may be short, requiring frequent dosing and potentially leading to low patient compliance and suboptimal therapeutic outcome.

e. Uptake of a drug through the mucosal membranes may be due to passive diffusion or by receptor-mediated active transport mechanisms.

7. **Indicate which one of the following statements is not correct:**

a. Delayed-release dosage forms can be defined as systems formulated to release the active ingredient at a time other than immediately after administration.

b. Colon-specific dosage forms are developed for the treatment of local and systemic diseases in the colon, including colorectal cancer and Crohn's disease.

c. In the plasma concentration versus time profile of a delayed-release oral dosage form C_{max} (but not T_{max}) is strongly dependent on the gastric emptying times.

d. Delayed-release systems can be used to protect the drug from degradation in the low-pH environment of the stomach.

e. Delayed-release systems can be used to protect the stomach from irritation by the drug.

8. **Indicate which one of the following statements is not correct:**

a. The release kinetics of the drugs from sustained-release matrix systems often follows a first-order kinetics.

b. The release kinetics of the drugs from sustained-release reservoir systems often follows a zero-order kinetics.

c. If the release of the drug from the dosage form is sustained such that the release takes place throughout the entire gastrointestinal tract, one can reduce C_{max} and prolong the time interval of drug concentration in the therapeutic range.

d. The use of sustained-release dosage forms may reduce the frequency of dosing, for example from three times a day to once a day.

e. Sustained-release dosage forms can achieve their release characteristics by the use of suitable polymers.

9. **Indicate which one of the following statements is not correct:**

a. In contrast to sustained-release forms, controlled-release systems are designed to lead to predictable and constant plasma concentrations, independently of the biological environment of the application site.

b. Controlled-release systems are controlling the drug concentration in the body, not just the release of the drug from the dosage form.

c. Controlled-release systems are used in a variety of administration routes, including transdermal, oral and vaginal administration.

d. In contrast to sustained-release forms, in controlled-release systems the dose is of less importance than the release rate from the therapeutic system.

e. Controlled-release systems are target-specific, which means they 'exclusively' deliver the drug to the target organ inside the body.

10. **Indicate which one of the following statements is not correct:**

a. In drug absorption, passive diffusion involves the diffusion of drugs across the cell membrane and is driven by a concentration gradient, with drugs moving from high to low concentration.

b. Carrier-mediated transport involves specific carrier proteins present in the cell membranes and can act either with a concentration gradient (facilitated diffusion) or against a concentration gradient (active absorption).

c. Endocytosis involves internalisation of substances by engulfment by the cell membrane which forms membrane-based vesicles within the cell, known as liposomes.

d. Some drugs can cross epithelia through gaps between the cells. This route is governed by passive diffusion and small hydrophilic molecules can pass through these gap junctions.

e. Drugs that are subjected to efflux processes include cytotoxic drugs such as taxol, steroids, immunosuppressants and antibiotics.

Further reading

Pharmaceutical dosage forms

Aulton ME (2007) *Aulton's Pharmaceutics – The Design and Manufacture of Medicines*. Edinburgh: Churchill Livingstone.

Florence AT, Attwood D (2008) *FASTtrack: Physicochemical Principles of Pharmacy*. London: Pharmaceutical Press.

Jones D (2008) *FASTtrack: Pharmaceutics: Dosage Form and Design*. London: Pharmaceutical Press.

Pharmacokinetics

Tozer TN, Rowland M (2006) *Introduction of Pharmacokinetics and Pharmacodynamics: The Quantitative Basis of Drug Therapy*. Baltimore, MD: Lippincott Williams & Wilkins.

chapter 2

Immediate-release drug delivery systems I: increasing the solubility and dissolution rate of drugs

Overview

In this chapter we will:

- describe the properties of an immediate-release drug delivery system
- discuss various strategies to improve solubility and dissolution rate of drugs at the:
  - molecular level, using co-solvents, salts, prodrugs and cyclodextrins
  - colloidal level, using lipid systems, emulsions and microemulsions
  - particulate level, by controlling the crystallinity, particle size and morphology of the drug
- describe methods to measure dissolution.

Introduction

Immediate-release drug delivery systems are designed to give a fast onset of drug action. Most drugs act through interaction with receptors in the body and, as this is a molecular interaction, drugs need to be molecularly dispersed, i.e. in solution. Therefore the solubility of a drug is a key consideration in drug formulation. Following on from this, if a solid dosage form is employed, dissolution is required so that the drug is released. Finally if absorption across epithelial barriers or cell membranes is required, the drug must be able to cross these biological barriers so it must have appropriate permeability. Within this chapter we will consider drug delivery strategies to improve drug solubility and dissolution as in many cases this will improve both the rate and extent of drug absorption.

KeyPoints

- Immediate-release systems aim to achieve a high plasma concentration quickly.
- For immediate release, drug solubility and dissolution are of the utmost importance.

KeyPoints

- Both solubility and dissolution are key factors controlling drug release from delivery systems. This can subsequently influence drug bioavailability.
- Many new drugs have low solubility due to their high crystallinity or increased lipophilicity.

Improving drug delivery by increasing the solubility and dissolution rate of the drug

Solubility is the ability of a solute (in our context, this will usually be the drug) to dissolve in a solvent (this can be water, a buffer solution or any other solvent, including so-called biorelevant media which are designed to mimic in vivo conditions in the gastrointestinal tract). Saturation solubility is the maximum solubility of the solute in the particular solvent at equilibrium conditions. Saturation solubility depends on temperature and pressure. For ionisable substances it is also affected by the pH of the solvent.

Whilst solubility is a thermodynamic property, dissolution is a kinetic property. The dissolution rate describes the speed with which a drug dissolves in a solvent. The dissolution rate depends not only on the type of solvent and temperature, but also on many other factors such as the size and surface area of the solid, mixing or stirring conditions and volume of the solvent.

As we have seen in Chapter 1, the bioavailability of a drug depends on its solubility and ability to cross biological membranes (permeability). Unfortunately, many modern drugs have low aqueous solubility. When given orally a dosage form in the gastrointestinal tract is still outside the body. The drug has to go into solution in the gastrointestinal tract to be able to cross the mucosal membrane to enter the body. The mechanism for overcoming the mucosal barrier can be by passive diffusion or it can involve active transport through interactions with transporter proteins. These processes take place on the molecular level, i.e. they require the drug to be dissolved. This means the drug in the dosage form must also have a sufficiently high dissolution rate. For example, in an oral dosage form if a drug has a reasonably high solubility but dissolves very slowly, sufficient drug concentrations cannot be achieved in the time the dosage form is present in the gastrointestinal tract.

Factors thought to be contributing to the trend of low solubility in new chemical entities include:

- Increased lipophilicity: many modern drugs are lipophilic. Such drug molecules are sometimes termed 'grease ball molecules'. They often have low melting points and low water solubility but show a fairly high solubility in lipophilic media.

Tip

Solubility can be predicted by comparing the solubility parameters of the two components (solute and solvent molecules). The solubility parameter is the square root of the cohesive energy density (the sum of the attractive forces between molecules). The cohesive energy density is the energy required to separate the molecules of a condensed phase (in our case a solid phase) to an infinite distance, where there is no longer an attractive force between them. The solubility parameter can be determined experimentally but more conveniently it can also be calculated from the molecular structure of the molecules.

■ Increased crystallinity: there is a trend for drugs to contain more functional groups and thus they are able to crystallise into very stable crystals having high melting points (frequently over 200 °C) with correspondingly low free energies. For these drugs a large amount of energy is necessary to free the molecules from the crystalline lattice. Strongly negative solvation energies are required for successfully dissolving these compounds. These drugs are often not particularly lipophilic, and therefore don't dissolve well in either water or oils. Sometimes these molecules are termed 'brick dust molecules'. These drugs may be termed 'solvophobic', to differentiate them from the above-mentioned lipophilic drugs.

It has been estimated that currently about one-third of novel chemical entities coming out of drug discovery research have an aqueous solubility of less than 10 µg/mL. Another third is between 10 and 100 µg/mL and the rest have a water solubility over 100 µg/mL. Even though the activity of modern drugs is usually very high, and thus only comparatively low plasma concentrations are needed to achieve the desired pharmacological effects, low water solubility is a major obstacle in developing effective drug delivery systems, especially for immediate-release dosage forms.

To address these problems various strategies to improve solubility, dissolution rate and the subsequent bioavailability of drugs have been developed by modifying the drug properties at the molecular level, by using colloidal drug delivery systems or by modifying the properties of drugs at the particulate level.

Improving the solubility of drugs on the molecular level

The options to improve solubility, dissolution rate and subsequent bioavailability of drugs at the molecular level include:

- using co-solvents
- using salt forms of drugs
- using prodrugs
- using cyclodextrins.

KeyPoints

- Drug solubility can be improved by dissolving the drug in a water co-solvent mixture.
- Drugs may precipitate upon co-solvent dilution.

Improving the solubility of drugs using co-solvents

If a drug has poor aqueous solubility, changing the solvent to a water-miscible organic solvent or a mixture of this solvent with water (then termed a co-solvent) is one option to improve its solubility. Generally solvents containing a hydroxyl group such as ethanol, propylene glycol, glycerol and poly(ethylene glycols) of varying molecular weights are used. This approach is often used in the formulation of oral pharmaceutical solutions.

However, to achieve a sufficiently high drug solubility in a water co-solvent mixture, the concentration of the co-solvent has to be quite high. Therefore, if the water-miscible co-solvent is diluted (for example, for an oral dosage form in the gastrointestinal fluids), the solubilisation power of the water co-solvent mixture can be rapidly lost and precipitation of the drug may occur. Also, high co-solvent concentrations may be unacceptable for parenteral formulations for toxicological reasons.

KeyPoints

- The formulation of drugs as salts can improve their solubility and dissolution.
- The choice of salt will depend on the pK_a of the drug, the route of administration and the dosage form.

Tip

It should be noted that a salt form of a drug not only influences its solubility and dissolution rate, but may also influence other properties of the drug that are important for the formulation of marketable drug delivery systems, such as its stability and processability (Chapter 1).

Tip

$pK_a = -\log_{10} K_a$, where K_a is the equilibrium constant for the dissociation of a weak acid.

Improving the solubility of drugs by salt formation

Formulation of drugs as salts instead of the use of the drug in its acid or base form is the most commonly used method to improve aqueous solubility and dissolution rate. To increase solubility by salt formation the pK_a values of the drug and the counterion have to be considered. To investigate the solubility increase upon salt formation, pH solubility curves have to be determined. These are schematically shown in Figure 2.1 for a basic drug (Figure 2.1a) and an acidic drug (Figure 2.1b), respectively. The counterion should have a pK_a that is sufficiently different from that of the drug. As a general rule, for acidic drugs the pK_a of the counterion should be higher by 2 pH values or more compared to the pK_a of the drug. For basic drugs, the pK_a of the counterion should be lower by 2 pH values or more compared to the pK_a of the drug. This is required as the counterion should bring the pH_{max} of the solution to values lower than the pH_{max} for basic drugs (Figure 2.1a) or higher than the pH for acidic drugs (Figure 2.1b).

It has been estimated that, of 300 new drugs approved by the US Food and Drug Administration (FDA) over the last 12 years, more than one-third have been salts, and the main reason for formulating these drugs as salts was to increase their aqueous solubility. Similarly, more than 50% of the drug monographs in the *United States Pharmacopeia* (USP 2006) are salt forms. Whilst it has been shown that in many cases the solubility of a salt is increased compared to the free acid or base form of the drug, the extent of this increase depends on the type of salt formed.

Usually in the salt selection process, the formulator prepares a range of salts and their physical and chemical properties have to be studied in detail to allow the most useful salt form to be selected. Properties of salt forms of drugs that have to be taken into account when deciding on a particular salt include chemical stability, hygroscopicity, polymorphism and mechanical properties.

Which salt form to employ also depends on the desired route of delivery and thus the dosage form or delivery systems to be used. A change of the salt form in the later stages of the formulation and development is costly in terms of money and time.

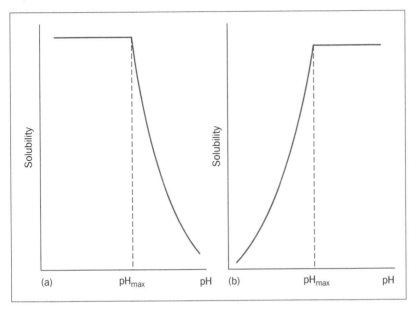

Figure 2.1 Idealised pH solubility profiles for: (a) a basic drug and (b) an acidic drug.

An important fact to take into consideration is that ions may not only be used to form the salt form of the drug but may also be present in the formulation for reasons other than salt formation. For example, calcium phosphate and sodium chloride are frequently used excipients for pharmaceutical dosage forms. On the other hand these ions may also be present in the biological environment of the drug, for example in the gastrointestinal tract. This can lead to an excessively high concentration of the counterion of the salt form, in turn leading to a decrease in the solubility of the drug. This is known as the common-ion effect.

However, depending on the pK_a and intrinsic solubility of the drug, it may not always be possible to form salts. Taking into account that solubility is often extremely low for modern drugs, other ways to improve solubility and dissolution rate of drugs need to be found for many compounds. Despite this, salt formation remains the main tool to increase solubility of poorly water-soluble drugs, and is thus often required in the formulation of an immediate-release dosage form.

The following ions are frequently used in salt formation (in decreasing order, according to the USP 2006 drug monographs):

- Anions: hydrochloride, sulphate, acetate, phosphate, chloride, maleate, mesylate
- Cations: sodium, potassium, calcium, aluminium.

Hydrochlorides and sodium salts are the salt formers that are most often used, as they have a comparatively low molecular weight (and thus add little to the overall mass of the dose of a salt compared to the free base or acid), and low toxicity.

KeyPoints

- Prodrugs are compounds which are converted by a chemical or enzymatic reaction into the active form of the drug.
- Prodrugs can be used to improve drug solubility by changing the drug molecule to a prodrug with higher water solubility.
- For drugs with high melting points it is also possible to increase their bioavailability by changing the parent drug into a prodrug with higher lipophilicity, leading to better membrane permeability.

Improving the solubility of drugs by prodrug design

Prodrugs are compounds which have to undergo biotransformation before exhibiting a biological response. They may then be further metabolised to be inactivated and excreted. Prodrugs are designed from existing drugs for various reasons, including:

- to improve solubility
- to increase drug stability
- to achieve sustained drug release
- to mask the taste of a drug
- to enable site-specific drug delivery.

To improve solubility through prodrug design, functional groups that increase solubility are added to the drug molecule. These groups themselves are not pharmacologically active parts of the molecule and must be removed by the action of enzymes or through chemical reactions to regenerate the biologically active drug molecule (parent molecule) from the prodrug.

The general synthetic prodrug strategy for improving solubility is to increase the polarity of drugs. This can be achieved by the addition of functional groups such as phosphate groups and sulfoxides. With phosphate groups, it is possible to convert the prodrug into a salt as the added groups are ionisable (anionic). Addition of an amine group allows the formation of hydrochloride salts, for example. The sulfoxide group on the other hand is non-ionisable.

Examples of two drugs in which this strategy has been used are given in Figure 2.2.

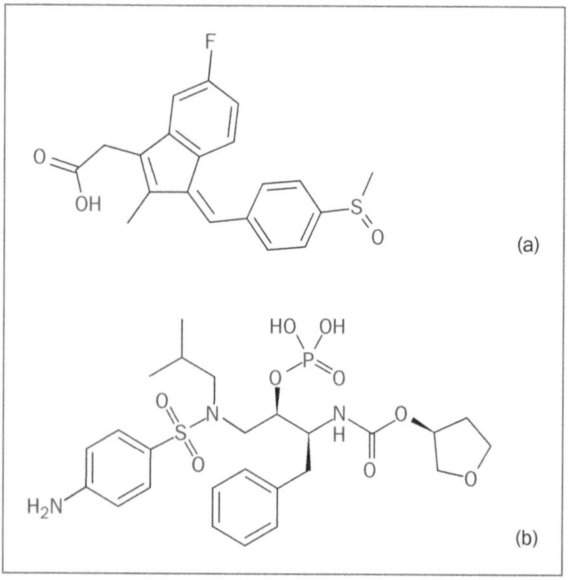

Figure 2.2 Chemical structures of two prodrug molecules used to improve solubility: (a) sulindac (containing a sulfoxide group as the prodrug functional group: the active form of the drug is sulindac sulfide); (b) fosamprenavir (containing a phosphate group as the prodrug functional group: the parent drug is amprenavir).

The addition of functional groups that make the parent molecule more hydrophilic may reduce drug absorption across mucosal membranes. For example, phosphate prodrugs need to be converted back to the parent molecule before absorption can take place. This may be achieved by the action of alkaline phosphatases in the apical brush border of the enterocytes in the gastrointestinal tract (Figure 2.3).

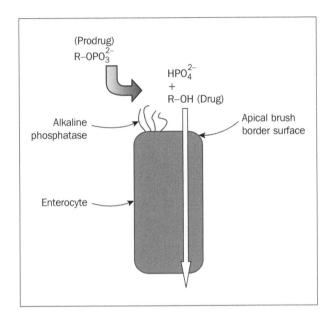

(Prodrug)
$R-OPO_3^{2-}$

HPO_4^{2-}
+
$R-OH$ (Drug)

Alkaline phosphatase

Apical brush border surface

Enterocyte

Figure 2.3 Schematic of the conversion of a phosphate prodrug to its parent drug molecule by alkaline phosphatase in the brush border.

For drugs with high melting points it is also possible to increase their bioavailability by changing the parent drug into a prodrug with higher lipophilicity. In these cases the aqueous solubility of the prodrug may be decreased compared to the parent compound. However, drug bioavailability is dependent on solubility and membrane permeability and a balance is often required. Even if the solubility of the prodrug in water is decreased, its solubilisation capacity in bile salt lecithin micelles present in the gastrointestinal tract may be increased and, due to the higher lipophilicity of the prodrug, absorption into the body may be increased.

It has to be kept in mind that increasing water solubility (or indeed bioavailability) of a prodrug is not the only change that may occur in the properties of a compound upon prodrug formation. Chemical stability, both in the solid state and in solution, may also be affected.

Tip

A prodrug is considered a novel chemical entity and therefore using prodrugs to improve a drug's solubility is costly and time-consuming as a new approval process is required. However, for existing drugs there is the possible advantage of prolonging the patent protection for the drug, if a new patent is granted for the prodrug. For new chemical entities, the decision to develop a prodrug further to improve aqueous solubility and bioavailability must be taken early at the developmental stage and requires extensive testing of parent compound and prodrug candidates.

Double esters

The introduction of more than one ester group is used for the delivery of the antibiotic cefuroxime axetil, the angiotensin-converting enzyme inhibitor fosinopril, and the AT_1-receptor antagonist candesartan cilexetil. In the case of candesartan cilexetil, intestinal esterases hydrolyse the double ester in an initial step, generating a hemiacetal which spontaneously decomposes to the pharmaceutical active free acid candesartan (Figure 2.4).

Figure 2.4 Conversion of the prodrug candesartan cilexetil to active form candesartan.

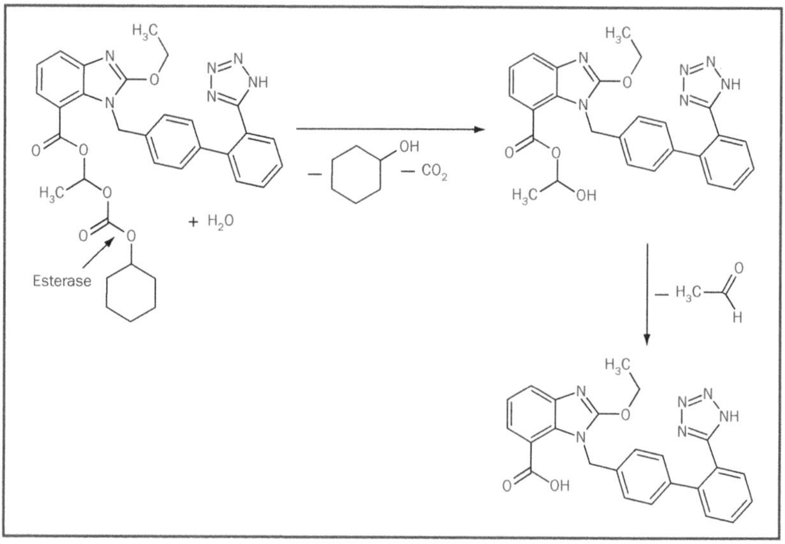

Tip

Prodrugs can also be used to mask the taste of drugs. The very bitter-tasting antibiotic chloramphenicol, for example, is esterified with palmitinic acid. Chloramphenicol palmitate is poorly soluble in the saliva, thereby avoiding the perception of bitterness. Pancreatic lipases then release the water-soluble chloramphenicol in the intestine by cleavage of the ester bond.

Improving the solubility of drugs by cyclodextrin complexation

Cyclodextrins are cyclic molecules derived from starch. Chemically, they are oligosaccharides containing six or more α-D-glucopyranose units linked by α-1,4 bonds. If the number of sugar units is six, they are termed α-cyclodextrins, if the number of sugar units is seven, they are called β-cyclodextrins, and if it is eight they are known as γ-cyclodextrins (Figure 2.5).

It is their molecular shape that makes cyclodextrins interesting excipients to increase the solubility of poorly water-soluble drugs by complexation. Cyclodextrins have a truncated cone shape (like a flowerpot without a bottom: Figure 2.5). Due to the orientation of the primary and secondary hydroxyl groups of the sugar units on the outside, the cyclodextrin molecule is hydrophilic on the outside. However, on the inside of the cone the molecule is less hydrophilic with carbons and the

Figure 2.5 Chemical structures of α-cyclodextrin (α-CD), β-cyclodextrin (β-CD) and γ-cyclodextrin (γ-CD) and shape of the γ-CD molecule.

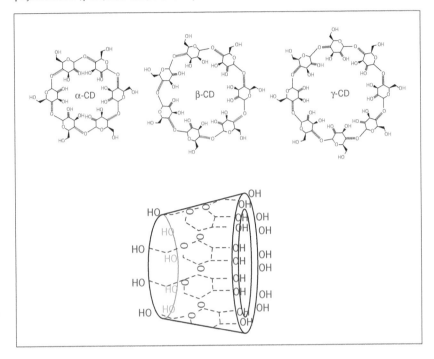

acetal group of the sugar units predominantly being located here and the polarity of the inside of the cavity is comparable to that of an ethanol solution. This local environment is favourable for complexation of poorly water-soluble drugs, hence improving their solubility. Another important criterion for the formation of a stable drug–cyclodextrin complex is that the cyclodextrin cavity is able to incorporate the size of the poorly water-soluble compound.

Besides the use of unmodified cyclodextrins, several derivatives of these molecules have also been synthesised, including a hydroxypropyl and a sulfobutylether derivative. The reason for these modifications is that these derivatives show a higher water solubility than the underivatised cyclodextrins, especially β-cyclodextrin. This may appear counterintuitive, as the replacement of a hydroxyl group on the sugar units may lead to a lower hydrophilicity of the molecule. However, it also means that the ability of these cyclodextrins to form intermolecular hydrogen bonds and thus to crystallise is reduced, which in turn increases their water solubility.

KeyPoints

- Cyclodextrins are truncated cone-shaped oligosaccharides.
- Poorly soluble drugs can be complexed within the cyclodextrin cavity to improve solubility and dissolution rate.

Tip

An acetal group has two single-bonded oxygens bonded to a carbon.

The complexation of drugs in the cavity of the cyclodextrins not only leads to an increase in the apparent solubility of the drug but also increases the dissolution rate. The dissolution rate of a drug may be described by the Noyes–Whitney equation. As the saturation solubility of the drug is increased by complexation it follows that its dissolution rate is also increased, as the dissolution rate is proportional to the saturation solubility. Thus cyclodextrin complexes of drugs can be used to formulate poorly water-soluble drugs as solutions (including oral solutions, intravenous and intramuscular parenteral solutions, and eye drops) but also as solid oral dosage forms (including tablets and capsules). More than 30 formulations containing drug–cyclodextrin complexes have been successfully introduced to the markets in Europe, the USA and Japan.

In order to form useful drug–cyclodextrin complexes their complexation constant should be determined by performing a phase solubility analysis. The higher the complexation constant, the less cyclodextrin is needed to complex the drug.

Phase solubility analysis

To assess complexation an excess of the poorly water-soluble drug is placed into vials containing a similar amount of solvent (usually water). To these suspensions increasing amounts of the cyclodextrin are added and the resulting suspensions are shaken or stirred for prolonged periods of time until equilibrium has been reached. They are then filtered (to remove excess solid drug) and the drug concentration is determined in the filtrate. In the resulting phase solubility diagrams the molar concentration of dissolved drug (drug in the filtrate which may be molecularly dispersed or complexed in the cyclodextrin) is plotted versus the molar cyclodextrin concentration, as shown in Figure 2.6. Note that the intercept with the y-axis is the saturation solubility of the uncomplexed drug. The shape of the resulting curves depends on the stoichiometry of the complex. A straight line with a slope of unity indicates formation of a 1:1 cyclodextrin–drug complex. A slope higher than unity indicates formation of higher-order complexes with respect to the drug (e.g. formation of a 1:2 cyclodextrin–drug complex) and, in contrast, a slope lower than unity indicates formation of higher-order complexes with respect to the cyclodextrin (e.g. formation of a 2:1 cyclodextrin–drug complex). Deviations from a linear slope indicate that initially one type of complex (e.g. a 1:1 complex) is formed but at higher cyclodextrin concentrations, higher-order complexes with respect to the drug or the cyclodextrin have formed.

The complexation constant for a drug–cyclodextrin complex can be calculated from the phase solubility curves using the following equation:

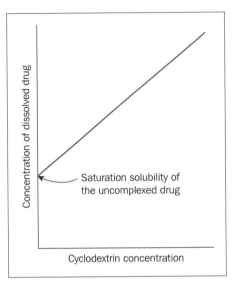

Figure 2.6 Schematic of a phase solubility diagram. A slope of 1 indicates formation of a 1:1 cyclodextrin to drug complex.

Complexation constant = slope of the curve/
(saturation solubility of the uncomplexed
drug × (1−slope of the curve))

From a practical formulation viewpoint, it should be noted that at higher cyclodextrin concentrations the cyclodextrins or the drug–cyclodextrin complexes may associate to form larger complexes that could precipitate. It is also possible that some drugs associate with the cyclodextrins in other ways than by inclusion into the cyclodextrin cavity. Additives to the formulation, such as cellulose derivatives and poly(vinylpyrrolidone) may also have pronounced effects on the complex formation. The drug–cyclodextrin complexation is an exothermic event, indicating that the complexation is enthalpy-driven, not entropy-driven. This is in contrast to the formation of micelles, for example, which is usually entropy-driven.

Improving the solubility of drugs on the colloidal level

It is also possible to improve dissolution and solubility of drugs on the *colloidal level* by solubilising the drug in colloidal systems, including:

- submicron emulsions
- microemulsions.

Colloids can be defined as particles in the nanometre size range (usually in the size range between approximately 10 and 500 nm). Colloids are either formed by dispersion of much larger particles (for example, coarse micrometre-sized particles in liquid dispersion) or they consist of associations of smaller molecules into larger colloidal particles, such as micelles and liposomes.

If the dispersions containing colloidal particles are thermodynamically stable (for example, a macromolecule solution, a micellar solution or a microemulsion) they are termed colloidal solutions. If the size of the dispersed particles is in the nanometre range but they are only kinetically stable, the resulting dispersions are termed colloidal dispersions (for example, submicron emulsions and liposome dispersions). The colloidal dispersions tend to coalesce or aggregate to reduce the total surface area of the dispersed particles which in turn reduces the surface free energy of the dispersed system.

Most pharmaceutically used colloidal formulations are based on lipids. Lipids are a diverse group of compounds, and examples include triglycerides, phospholipids and cholesterol.

Tip

If the dispersed particles are in the micrometre size range we can term these dispersions *coarse dispersions*. They are not thermodynamically stable. Emulsions and suspensions are examples of pharmaceutically used coarse dispersions.

KeyPoints

- Lipids can be classified according to their ability to interact with water.
- Class I polar lipids include long- and medium-chain triglycerides.
- Class II polar lipids include lecithin and monoglycerides.
- Class III polar lipids include surfactants and bile salts.

Lipid classification

There are various types of lipids employed in formulations, and they can be classified physicochemically according to their ability to interact with water.

1. Non-polar lipids are insoluble in water and do not form a monolayer on the water–air interface. Pharmaceutically the most important example of this lipid class is paraffin, a mixture of aliphatic hydrocarbons.
2. Polar lipids can be further subdivided into three classes:
    a. Class I polar lipids are insoluble and non-swelling lipids. Like non-polar lipids they do not (or only very sparingly) dissolve in water. They do, however, spread on the air–water interface to form stable monolayers. Class I lipids commonly used are vegetable oils (long-chain triglycerides) such as corn oil, olive oil and rape seed oil. These can be hydrogenated to reduce oxidative degradation. Medium-chain triglycerides such as coconut oil or palm seed oil are also used.
    b. Class II polar lipids are insoluble and swelling lipids. Like class I lipids they form monolayers on the air–water interface and are practically insoluble in water. In contrast to class I molecules,

Figure 2.7 Schematic of lyotropic liquid crystalline structures: (a) lamellar; (b) hexagonal; (c) cubic lyotropic liquid crystals.

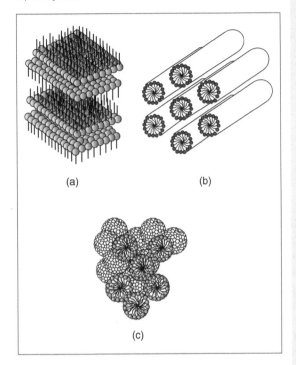

(a)   (b)

(c)

Tips

Swelling lipids usually have a crystalline or liquid crystalline layered structure and are able to incorporate water between their layers, leading to a swelling of the crystalline or liquid crystalline structures.

Liquid crystals
This is a state of matter, between the crystalline solid state and the liquid state. It has been estimated that about 5% of organic molecules are able to exist in this state. Liquid crystals have some properties of crystalline solids, such as long-range order of the molecules in some dimensions, and some properties of liquids, such as random orientation in other dimensions.

Lyotropic liquid crystals
These form upon addition of a solvent (most commonly water) to a solid. Depending on the arrangements of the molecules in the lyotropic liquid, crystal, lamellar, hexagonal and cubic phases can be differentiated. For example, lamellar liquid crystals have long-range order in one dimension and hexagonal liquid crystals have long-range order in two dimensions (Figure 2.7).

they do however swell in water (above a certain temperature) to form lyotropic liquid crystals, such as lamellar, cubic and hexagonal phases.

Pharmaceutically relevant examples of this lipid class are lecithin derivatives (such as phosphatidylcholine and phosphatidylethanolamine) and monoglycerides of fatty acids.

c. Class III polar lipids are soluble amphiphilic molecules (also termed surfactants). These molecules spread on the air–water interface but form unstable monolayers. They also show some molecular solubility in water below the critical micelle-forming concentration (CMC). At concentrations higher than the CMC they form micelles (association colloids).

Class III polar lipids can be further subdivided into class IIIa and class IIIb polar lipids, depending on their ability to form liquid crystals in higher concentration in water (class IIIa polar lipids do form liquid crystals; class IIIb polar lipids do not).

Pharmaceutically relevant examples of these lipids are anionic, non-ionic and cationic surfactants (class IIIa) and free and conjugated bile salts (class IIIb).

KeyPoints

- Lipid mixtures can be used to dissolve poorly water-soluble, lipophilic drugs and can be delivered in soft gelatine capsules.
- Digestion within the gastrointestinal tract of class I polar lipids improves drug absorption.
- Self-emulsifying systems increase bioavailability of orally administered lipophilic, poorly water-soluble drugs.

Lipid-based, water-free formulations

Lipid-based drug delivery systems are an effective way of improving the solubility of lipophilic drugs. Examples of such formulations are:

- lipid solutions
- self-emulsifying drug delivery systems.

The simplest formulation of this type is to dissolve the drug in an oil (class I polar lipid), such as medium-chain triglycerides or vegetable oils and to load this formulation into a soft gelatin capsule. For a drug to be dissolved in a class I polar lipid solvent it has to be lipophilic, thus 'grease ball' molecules are suitable, whereas 'brick dust' molecules often cannot be dissolved at a concentration required to formulate a lipid solution to achieve the required dose.

These formulations are solutions of the drug in the lipid, so the drug does not form a colloidal but rather a molecular dispersion. However, after oral delivery, the lipid triglycerides will be subjected to lipolysis in the gastrointestinal tract, forming two fatty acids and one monoglyceride in the process. These molecules combined with bile salts and lecithin present in the gastrointestinal tract can now solubilise the lipophilic drug in micelles to form a micellar (i.e. colloidal) dispersion. Uptake of the drug into the body may then occur either by partitioning of the drug into the cells of the gastric mucosa or possibly also by uptake of the micelles.

Therefore formulations of drugs dissolved in oils (class I polar lipids) require micellisation to take place in the intestine with the help of lipases, bile salts and lecithin. Alternatively, surfactants (class IIIa polar lipids) can be added to the oil formulation. This can lead to a water-free formulation which, upon addition of water in the gastrointestinal tract, 'spontaneously', i.e. without the input of large amounts of energy, can form colloidal dispersions which can be either submicron emulsions or even microemulsions. Such systems are called self-emulsifying drug delivery systems (SEDDS) or self-microemulsifying drug delivery systems (SMEDDS), depending on the type of colloidal dispersion or colloidal solution formed.

Formulation of lipophilic drugs in SEDDS or SMEDDS has two potential advantages:

1. Slightly less lipophilic but still poorly water-soluble drugs may be dissolved in these formulations.
2. The formulation can form submicron emulsions or even microemulsions by being diluted with water in the gastrointestinal tract independent of the activity of bile salts and

lecithin which, depending on the state of the patient, may be present at differing concentrations in the gastrointestinal tract.

Therefore these systems improve absorption of drugs from the gastrointestinal tract and reduce food effects which may lead to unpredictable absorption.

Class IIIa lipids used to formulate SEDDS and SMEDDS include surfactants such as Cremophor EL, Tween, Span, Labrafil, Labrasol, Gelucire, TPGS and others.

In some cases no class I polar lipid at all may be added to the drug. In these cases the solution of the drug in the formulation is achieved by adding large amounts of class IIIa lipids together with water-miscible co-solvents such as propylene glycol or poly(ethylene glycol). Whilst these systems have a good solvent capacity for drugs that are less soluble in strongly lipophilic formulations, care must be taken to avoid precipitation of the drug as the co-solvent is diluted in the gastrointestinal tract.

Emulsions and microemulsions

Emulsions are two-phase systems, containing an oil phase and a water phase, one of them being a continuous and the other being a dispersed phase. Depending on which phase is the dispersed phase, emulsions can be differentiated into water-in-oil and oil-in-water emulsions. The particle size of the droplets of the dispersed phase may vary and can be in the micrometre (coarse) or nanometre (colloidal) range. The latter are called submicron emulsions. Due to the oil phase of the formulation, lipophilic drugs can be solubilised to improve their delivery.

Emulsions are thermodynamically unstable, i.e. for their formation usually a high amount of energy is required and has to be provided by mixing, shaking or sonication. Even if these systems form 'spontaneously' in the gastrointestinal tract, they remain thermodynamically unstable, as

Tip

The fed or fasted state of a person can significantly influence the bioavailability of low-solubility drugs. Co-administration of drugs with food often provides better solubilising conditions in the gastrointestinal tract since lipases and bile salt production are stimulated by food.

Tip

To formulate SEDDS or SMEDDS the phase behaviour of class I polar lipid–class IIIa polar lipid–water mixtures needs to be determined. Ternary-phase diagrams should be constructed to detect the solubility of the drug in question in the various phases that may form upon dilution of the lipid mixture with water.

KeyPoints

- Emulsions are two-phase systems containing oil and a water phase. Poorly soluble drugs can be solubilised within the oil phase of the formulation to improve their delivery.
- Emulsions are thermodynamically unstable due to the interfacial tension between the oil and water phase and their large interfacial area.
- Microemulsions are thermodynamically stable colloidal solutions containing suitable mixtures of oil, water, and surfactant(s) and co-surfactant(s).

the interfacial area between the oil and the water phase increases due to the dispersion of the droplets. This results in a high surface free energy (G_s) of the systems as G_s depends on the interfacial tension (γ) between the phases and the interfacial area between the phases (A): $G_s = \gamma A$. Even though the addition of suitable surfactants as emulsifiers lowers the interfacial tension (and thus kinetically stabilises the dispersion), γ remains to be a positive value and thus the surface free energy is increased as one phase is dispersed in the other. To lower its surface free energy, the dispersed droplets aggregate, often followed by coalescence as this leads to a reduction of the interfacial area.

This thermodynamic instability of emulsions may be a problem in their application. Emulsions are most commonly used for oral and topical administration. After oral administration, oil droplets are digested by the lipases and the resulting partial glycerides and fatty acids are subjected to bile salt micellisation. However, these processes are prevalent mainly in the small intestine and not in the stomach. Also the activity of lipases and solubilisers may vary from patient to patient and depends on the fasting state of the patient.

Emulsions may also be formulated to have droplet sizes small enough and stabilities high enough to allow intravenous administration, for example for parenteral nutrition. These intravenous emulsions can also be used for drug delivery, e.g. Diazemuls is used to deliver diazepam parenterally.

Physically, *microemulsions* are one-phase systems, more closely related to micellar solutions than to coarse emulsions. Microemulsions are thus thermodynamically stable colloidal solutions, unlike emulsions. They are formed by suitable mixtures of oils (class I polar lipids), water and surfactants (class IIIa polar lipids). Due to their class I lipid component they can be used to deliver poorly water-soluble drugs. Either a combination of several surfactants is used or water-miscible co-solvents (such as ethanol or glycerol) are added to the formulation. If no co-solvent is added, often the oil–surfactant–water mixtures result in the formation of liquid crystals at higher surfactant or water concentrations, such as lamellar, hexagonal and cubic liquid crystals. Therefore, by determining the phase diagram of the components it is necessary to identify combinations that result in the formation of microemulsions. Microemulsions often form spontaneously by simply mixing the individual components.

Several types of microemulsions can be differentiated. Droplet-type microemulsions contain nanometre-sized oil or water droplets and are usually called water-in-oil or

Tip

The name 'microemulsion' is somewhat misleading as microemulsions are neither emulsions nor do they contain dispersed droplets in the micrometre size range. However, the name is established and used widely.

oil-in-water microemulsions, depending on the nature of the droplets. As these droplets do not form a separate phase they are sometimes termed oil or water pseudophase. As the oil-in-water microemulsion type contains a class I polar lipid component they are also sometimes termed 'swollen micellar solutions', in which the surfactant forms micelles into which the oil is solubilised, which leads to a swelling of the micelle. Similarly, water-in-oil microemulsions are sometimes termed 'swollen inverse micellar solutions', in which the surfactant forms an inverse micelle into which the water is solubilised. Some combinations of oil, water, surfactant (usually a mixture of several surfactants) and co-solvent can form microemulsion systems spanning from very low to very high water concentrations in the phase diagram. These systems are called balanced microemulsions. For such systems, between the water-in-oil microemulsion and the oil-in-water microemulsion regions in the phase diagram, one frequently finds so-called bicontinuous microemulsion in which the oil and water pseudophase are intimately intertwined and separated by a surfactant monolayer. The different types of microemulsions are schematically represented in Figure 2.8.

Tip

Microemulsions are thermodynamically stable (unlike submicron emulsions) because the interfacial tension between the droplets and the continuous liquid is reduced to extremely low values. However, as it remains positive, low interfacial tension cannot be the only reason why microemulsions are thermodynamically stable. In addition, microemulsion droplets are not static but form, fall apart and reform, and the surfactant molecules are constantly exchanged between the droplets. These processes occur in the nanosecond time scale. Thus there is a large entropy of mixing which overcomes the positive enthalpy of the increased interfacial area to result in an overall negative free energy for microemulsion formation.

Figure 2.8 Schematic representation of a water-in-oil microemulsion (left), a bicontinuous microemulsion (middle) and an oil-in-water microemulsion (right).

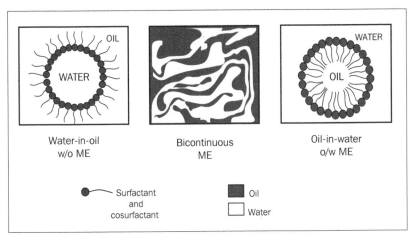

OIL

WATER

Water-in-oil
w/o ME

Bicontinuous
ME

WATER

OIL

Oil-in-water
o/w ME

Surfactant
and
cosurfactant

Oil

Water

Neoral, a self-microemulsifying ciclosporin formulation

The cyclic peptide ciclosporin is an effective immunosuppressant used extensively in organ transplantation. Chemically it consists of 11 amino acids and has a molecular weight of just over 1200. Ciclosporin has a very low water solubility but possesses a fairly good solubility in vegetable oils and ethanol. The original drug formulation was an emulsion preconcentrate delivered in a soft gelatin capsule. This formulation formed a coarse dispersion (emulsion) in the gastrointestinal tract after breakdown of the capsule in the stomach. Absorption of the drug occurred after solubilisation of the oil droplets by the action of lipases, bile salts and lecithin. Using this emulsion preconcentrate an acceptable bioavailability of approximately 30% could be achieved. However it was found that this bioavailability could vary between 10% and 60% in individual patients. This was because the drug is mainly absorbed from the mixed micelles formed in the gastrointestinal tract, but this process of micellisation is variable in patients depending on the bile salt concentration in the small intestine (which is where the drug is absorbed). This is a frequent problem in liver transplant patients.

The original formulation (called Sandimmune) was thus reworked with the aims to improve the bioavailability of the drug and to reduce the variability in bioavailability. This was achieved by replacing the emulsion preconcentrate with a microemulsion preconcentrate. The new formulation (called Neoral) leads to a dispersion of the drug in the gastrointestinal tract after opening of the soft gelatin capsule to microemulsion droplets of less than 50 nm in diameter. Importantly, this dispersion is achieved independently of the action of lipases, bile salts or lecithin.

The original ciclosporin formulation contained corn oil (a class I polar lipid) and the class IIIa polar lipid Labrafil M 2125 CS (polyoxyethylated glycolysed glycerides) as emulsifier. Replacing these components with corn oil mono-ditriglycerides and polyoxyl 40 hydrogenated castor oil (both class IIIa polar lipids) and adding propylene glycol as a co-solvent, the formulation could be reworked into a SMEDDS.

Improving the solubility of drugs on the particulate level

For drugs of the 'brick dust' type, formulation into lipidic systems is less of an option compared with the 'grease ball' type. However it is also possible to modify the properties of these types of molecules at the level of the drug particle, by crystallising the drug in a metastable polymorphic form, by converting the crystalline structure of the drug particles into an amorphous form or by changing particle size and particle morphology.

Improving drug solubility and dissolution rate by decreasing particle size and changing particle morphology

The Noyes–Whitney equation links the dissolution rate of a drug to its saturation solubility and to the surface area of the drug particles.

$$\text{Dissolution rate} = \frac{dX}{dt} = \frac{AD}{h}\left(C_s - \frac{X_t}{V}\right)$$

where:

- A is the surface area of the particle
- D is the diffusivity (diffusion constant) of the molecule
- h is the effective boundary layer thickness around the dissolving particle
- C_s is the saturation solubility of the drug
- X_t is the amount of drug dissolved at time t
- V is the volume of solvent available for dissolution.

From this equation we can see that, if a formulation process increases the saturation solubility of the drug (C_s), it increases the dissolution rate. However, increasing the surface area of the drug particles also increases the dissolution rate. The total surface area for a given mass or volume of particles (known as the mass or volume-specific surface area, respectively) increases if the particle size is reduced. Therefore reducing the particle size of a drug powder (for example, in a milling process) increases the dissolution rate of the drug. In the dynamic situation of the gastrointestinal tract, a high dissolution rate should lead to higher bioavailability if drug solubility and not drug absorption is the rate-limiting step.

Reducing the particle size also decreases the effective boundary layer thickness around the dissolving particles, further improving dissolution rate. In the case of very small particles (in the low nanometre size range) not only the dissolution rate but also the saturation solubility may be increased. For spherical particles the following equation can be applied:

$$\log \frac{S}{S_0} = \frac{2\gamma M}{2.303 r \rho RT}$$

where:

- S is the saturation solubility of the drug
- S_0 is the saturation solubility of an infinitively large particle of the drug (infinitively here means particles in the micrometre size range)

KeyPoints

- Drug dissolution can also be improved by the reduction of the drug particle size.
- This is because increasing the surface area of the drug particles increases the dissolution rate.
- Particle size reduction can be achieved by milling processes and high-pressure homogenisation.
- Surfactants and polymers can be used to reduce particle aggregation in these processes.

- γ is the interfacial tension between the particle and the solvent
- M is the molecular weight of the drug
- r is the radius of the particle
- ρ is the density of the particle
- R is the gas constant
- T is the temperature.

Micronisation (i.e. reducing the drug particle size to the low micron range by milling techniques) has been applied in the pharmaceutical industry for many years. Milling techniques can now reduce the drug particle size to the nanometre size range.

Two techniques have been used to achieve nanosizing of drug particles: wet milling using bead mills and high-pressure homogenisation. In both processes particle size reduction is achieved in a dispersion fluid in which the drug is insoluble. After the size-diminishing process the dispersion fluid has to be removed, usually by fluid bed or spray drying. Particle sizes that currently can be achieved using nanosizing techniques range between 100 and 200 nm.

Nanosizing

Several medicines on the market use nanosizing technology with the aim of achieving higher bioavailability and reducing food effects (which can lead to erratic bioavailabilities depending on the fasting state of the patient). These products include:

- Rapamune, containing the immunosuppressant sirolimus
- Emend, containing the antiemetic aprepitant
- Tricor and Triglide, containing the antihypercholesterolaemia drug fenofibrate
- Megace ES, containing the appetite stimulant megesterol acetate.

For such small particle sizes one of the main problems is to keep the nanosized material as individual particles, in other words to avoid aggregation. If aggregation occurs, many of the advantages of the nanosized material may be lost. Aggregation is caused by the increase in surface free energy of the nanosized particles, due to their very high volume or mass specific surface areas. As discussed earlier, the interfacial free energy $G_i = A\gamma$, where γ is the interfacial tension between the particles and the surrounding phase and A is the surface area of the particles. Therefore non-aggregated particles can be retained by reducing the interfacial tension. This can be achieved by adding surfactants in the milling process. Non-ionic and anionic surfactants are used, including polysorbates, sodium dodecylsulphate and sodium docusate. The surfactants are adsorbed on to the newly formed surfaces with their polar head groups pointing towards the liquid phase. The use of ionic surfactants provides a charge on the particle surface and electrostatic repulsion between the particles, further reducing particle aggregation. Polymeric stabilisers can also be used instead of, or in combination with, surfactants. Cellulose derivatives such as hydroxypropylcellulose and hydroxypropylmethylcellulose, poly(vinylpyrrolidone) or pluronics (poly(ethylene glycol polypropylene glycol) block copolymers, a polymeric surfactant) are normally used. These polymers act mainly through steric stabilisation. Additionally, the surfactant and polymeric excipients also increase wetting of the drug particles, which is a necessary prerequisite for the dissolution process to occur.

Typical ratios of drug to surfactant or drug to polymer are in the range of 1:0.05 to 1:0.5 (w/w). If nanoparticles are further formulated into capsules and tablets it is also necessary to add re-dispersants, and here mainly sugars or sugar alcohols such as sucrose, lactose or mannitol are used.

During the size reduction process, conversion of the crystalline form of the drug into the amorphous state can occur. This may further increase dissolution rate and solubility of the drug (compared to the crystalline form; see section on improving drug solubility by using amorphous forms, below); however, it is usually not desired in the nanomilling process as it leads to particles that are physically unstable and they may convert back to the crystalline state during storage of the drug or medicine. Also, an unknown and variable amorphous content may lead to unpredictable bioavailability.

Besides decreasing the particle size, it is also possible to increase the dissolution rate by carefully controlling the crystallisation process, for example by using various solvents from which the drug is crystallised or by varying the crystallisation rate, for example through temperature modifications. This may lead to the formation of the same crystalline form of the drug but differences in the morphology of the resulting crystals. For example, phenytoin and dipyridamole can be crystallised from different solvents, resulting in either rod-like or rhombic crystals under certain conditions and needle-like crystals using other solvents. The shape of the crystals (like their size) influences the surface-to-volume ratio of the resulting particles. It could be shown that the needle-like crystals had a higher dissolution rate than crystals with other habits.

Tip

Steric stabilisation results from the hydrophilic chain of the polymers being highly hydrated. Close contact of particles causes these chains to overlap, resulting in loss of hydrating water and loss in conformational freedom. This subsequently causes the particles to be pushed apart.

Tip

Drugs in the amorphous state have a higher solubility and dissolution rate compared to their crystalline counterparts.

Improving drug solubility by using metastable polymorphs

Many pharmaceutical compounds can crystallise in different crystallographic forms. These are termed polymorphs. Polymorphs

KeyPoints

- Polymorphism is the ability of a solid to exist in more than one crystallographic form or crystal structure.
- The polymorphic form of a drug will influence its solubility.

Tip

The crystallographic form of a crystal has to be differentiated from the shape or habit of the crystalline particle. Whilst the crystallographic form refers to the specific arrangement, for example of the molecules of a drug in a crystalline lattice, the habit refers to the outer shape or appearance of the crystalline particles (e.g. needle, platelet or prism).

of a drug are chemically identical, but as they crystallise into different lattices, their physical properties, such as their density and solubility, may be different. Different polymorphic forms can be prepared by changing the crystallisation conditions. Most modern drugs show polymorphism, frequently being able to crystallise in three or more forms. Examples of drugs showing polymorphism include carbamazepine, sulfathiazole and saquinavir.

Solvent molecules may form part of the crystalline structure when they are included into the lattice during the crystallisation process from the solvent. The general expression for such crystals, containing drug and solvent molecules, is solvates. Examples include:

- Hydrates: water is incorporated into the crystalline lattice.
- Ethanolates: ethanol is incorporated into the crystalline lattice.

The incorporation of solvent molecules is usually stoichiometric, which means that monohydrates and dihydrates can be formed depending on the molar ratio of drug to water molecules in the crystal. Such forms are sometimes also termed pseudopolymorphs. In their own right solvates can show polymorphism.

At any given condition, only one polymorphic form of a drug is thermodynamically stable. However, other forms may be metastable, i.e. activation energy is required to convert the metastable form into the stable one. If the stability of the metastable form in high enough, crystallising a drug in this form and not the thermodynamically stable form is possible, and this may improve wetting, dissolution rate and the solubility of the compound. For example, using chloramphenicol palmitate in its metastable polymorphic form leads to a much higher bioavailability then using the thermodynamically stable form.

However, using a metastable form of a drug instead of the stable polymorph increases solubility usually by only two- or threefold and may not sufficiently increase bioavailability. Further, there is a risk that the metastable form may convert back to the stable form of the drug. This can occur in the final dosage form upon storage or upon administration of the drug, when the crystals are dispersed in the gastrointestinal tract. If the metastable form converts back to the stable form or converts to a hydrate in the gastrointestinal tract, the solubility advantage of the metastable form is lost. In general, hydrates have lower water solubilities than non-hydrate forms.

Improving drug solubility by using amorphous forms

Converting a crystalline drug particle into the amorphous state leads to increased solubility and dissolution rate. The amorphous state of a solid is characterised by the absence of long-range order in position and orientation of the drug molecules. By contrast, crystals show three-dimensional long-range positional and orientational order. Although amorphous materials lack long-range order, they may however show short-range order. For example, drugs containing carboxylic acid groups may form dimers through hydrogen bonding. The same has been reported for drugs containing amide groups such as carbamazepine.

A lack of long-range order is also typical for melts and solutions. In contrast to these, however, the amorphous state is practically solid or at least has a very high viscosity, and in practical terms does not flow, at least below the glass transition temperature (see below). This means that in simple terms, the amorphous state has the order of a melt but the appearance of a solid.

Producing the amorphous state

Figure 2.9 shows how the amorphous state can be generated. If a crystalline drug

KeyPoints

- The amorphous state is characterised by a lack of long-range order between drug molecules.
- Drugs in the amorphous state often have a high solubility and dissolution rate.
- Amorphous compounds can be produced by melting the drug and then cooling the melt at a rapid rate.
- Co-melting the drug with a polymer can be used to improve stability of the amorphous system.

Figure 2.9 Heating and cooling paths of a melt. T_m, melting temperature of the crystalline form; T_g, glass transition temperature of the amorphous form; T_k, Kautzmann temperature.

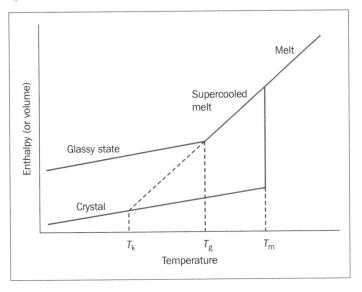

is heated a sharp change in many thermodynamic properties occurs at the melting point where the drug is transformed to a liquid melt. Whilst this process is generally reversible (if no chemical degradation takes place in the melt), if the melt is cooled sufficiently fast, it is possible to overrun the recrystallisation temperature, thus there is insufficient time for the drug molecules in the melt to orient themselves to form crystals. At temperatures below the melting point of the drug, a supercooled melt is formed. This state is also known as the rubbery state. In the rubbery state the supercooled melt still behaves like a highly viscous liquid and is likely to recrystallise to the thermodynamically stable crystal form during storage of the drug. However, if the temperature is further reduced, the gradient of change of the thermodynamic properties is altered in a certain temperature range. This temperature range is known as the glass transition temperature and marks the temperature when the rubbery state changes into the so-called glassy state. In this form the drug shows a fairly high resistance against recrystallisation, as the molecular motions of the molecules are now very low.

Tip

Depending on the cooling rate, the glass transition occurs at different temperatures. The slower the melt is cooled, the lower the glass transition temperature is. Theoretically the lowest temperature at which the glass transition can occur is the Kautzmann temperature (Figure 2.9). On the other hand, the slower the cooling rate, the higher is the likelihood that recrystallisation occurs from the rubbery state, and thus in practical terms high cooling rates are preferred to create glassy solids. Nevertheless the glass transition (unlike the melting point) is not a thermodynamic property but a kinetic event depending on the conditions at which it has been reached. Therefore it is not surprising that different values for glass transition temperatures of drugs are found in the literature.

With regard to the stability of a drug in the amorphous state it is important to consider the following:

- The glass transition temperature of an amorphous form should be higher than the storage temperature to achieve sufficient physical stability of the amorphous state against crystallisation.
- Water acts as a potent plasticiser, lowering the glass transition temperature of the drug substantially, even at low water concentrations.

Many amorphous systems are hygroscopic and avoiding water uptake is thus an important issue. One solution is to use only drugs with very high glass transitions (above 70–80 °C). Generally, for drugs to have a high glass transition temperature they also need a high melting point.

However, co-melting the drug with a (usually amorphous) polymer which has a high glass transition temperature can increase the overall glass transition of the mixture, resulting in a stabilised amorphous form of the drug. Moreover, using a hydrophilic polymer can improve wetting.

If the drug and the polymer form a single-phase amorphous system, this leads to a strong increase in solubility and dissolution rate of the drug because:

- No crystalline lattice energy needs to be overcome in the dissolution process.
- The drug has a maximally reduced drug particle size (in fact, reduced to a molecular dispersion).
- The water-soluble polymer is present in the glass solution in an intimate mixture with the drug.

General guidelines in the choice of an appropriate polymer and the drug:polymer ratio include:

- The polymer should have a strong antiplasticising effect. This means the glass transition temperature of the polymer should be high.
- It is usually advantageous if the drug and the polymer show some interactions, for example through hydrogen bonding, as this further reduces the mobility of the drug molecules and prevents them from crystallising.
- The drug and polymer should have a good mutual solubility in the solid state.

It is also possible to achieve the formation of glass solutions via a solution of drug and polymer in a common solvent and then remove the liquid by spray drying or the addition of an antisolvent (co-precipitation). Another technique employed to create glass solutions is melt extrusion. This process is commonly used in the polymer industry and has recently been applied in the pharmaceutical field. Melt extrusion combines melting the drug–polymer mixture with intensive shearing in an extrusion process using either single-screw or twin-screw extruders. In contrast to the solution-based techniques, no solvents are used, thus minimising the possibility of glass transition reductions due to residual solvent.

Within a glass solution, both components are in the amorphous state. However it is also possible that the drug may still be crystalline but finely dispersed in an amorphous matrix of the polymer (solid dispersion). In this case the drug dissolution rate increase is usually not as high as if drug and excipient form a one-phase glass solution. However, an advantage is that the drug is in a more stable state and thus physical and chemical stability of the formulation may be higher.

Polymers such as poly(vinylpyrrolidone) and cellulose derivatives such as hydroxypropylmethylcellulose (HPMC) and

Tip

A solution is a molecular dispersion and it is possible to have solid solutions. Generally, if drug and polymer have solubility parameters close to each other, they should be miscible. The larger the difference between the two solubility parameters, the more likely it is that drug and polymer will not form a solution, at least not over the entire range of binary mixtures.

hydroxypropylcellulose (HPC) are most often used to formulate drugs as glass solutions. Whilst poly(vinylpyrrolidone) is suitable for this process due to its amorphous nature, high glass transition temperature, ability to form hydrogen bonds with many drugs and suitable solubility parameter for many low-solubility drugs, it is very hygroscopic and much care must be taken to avoid moisture uptake of the formulation, for example by packaging of tablets into aluminium blisters. Comparably, cellulose derivatives are less hygroscopic.

Usually solid dispersions are further processed into capsules or tablets for oral administration. Several drugs have been marketed as glass solutions or solid dispersions, including:

- Kaletra tablets (containing a lopinavir and ritonavir combination with poly-(vinylpyrrolidone))
- Sporanox capsules (containing itraconazole with HPMC)
- Rezulin tablets (containing troglitazone with poly(vinylpyrrolidone))
- Certican tablets (containing everolimus with HPMC)
- ProGraf capsules (containg tacrolimus with HPMC)
- Nivadil tablets (containing nivaldipine with HPMC).

How to determine the dissolution rate of a drug

Dissolution testing is the standard method for measuring drug release from a solid dosage form. As the dissolution rate of a drug depends on the conditions under which the test is performed, the pharmacopoeias contain detailed descriptions of the test apparatuses for pure drug powders, tablets and capsules. These apparatuses and the test methods are described in great detail to allow reproducible measurements from day to day and from lab to lab. Typical dissolution tests include the intrinsic dissolution test (for pure drugs) and the use of the basket apparatus, the paddle apparatus and flow-through cells for tablets and capsules. Time limits for dissolution of a certain percentage of the dose of an individual drug formulated in an immediate-release dosage form are given in the monographs of the pharmacopoeias.

KeyPoints

- Dissolution tests ensure that dosage forms give reproducible and predictable release profiles in vitro.
- In vitro dissolution studies do not closely mimic in vivo conditions. Biorelevant dissolution media can be used to improve the tests.

These classical dissolution tests of the pharmacopoeias have to be seen as primarily pharmaceutical quality tests. This means the dissolution test ensures that the dosage forms produced have a reproducible and predictable behaviour in vitro and thus their manufacturing has to be within tightly specified limits to allow for reproducible and comparable results.

Importantly, whilst dissolution tests (carried out in so-called simulated gastric fluid and simulated intestinal fluid) may be related to the behaviour of the dosage form in vivo, the conditions used in these tests do not closely mimic the situation in vivo. If we want to use dissolution tests to predict the behaviour of the dosage form in vivo we need to mimic the in vivo situation more closely. To achieve this aim so-called biorelevant dissolution media have been developed to simulate the fasted and fed states.

Biorelevant dissolution media are used to predict the in vivo behaviour of the formulation mainly in the development process. Having fasted- and fed-state simulated fluids also allows the prediction of food effects on the dissolution and thus bioavailability of orally administered drugs. The use of biorelevant dissolution media may greatly influence and facilitate formulation optimisation.

Tips

A fasted-state simulated intestinal fluid (FaSSIF) may contain: sodium taurocholate 3 mmol/L, lecithin 0.75 mmol/L, NaOH (pellets) 0.174 g, $NaH_2PO_4 \cdot H_2O$ 1.977 g, NaCl 3.093 g, purified water to 500 mL. Such a fluid, containing a bile salt and a phospholipid, better reflects the situation in the small intestine in the fasted state, allowing for solubilisation of lipophilic drugs in the bile salt–lecithin mixed micelles.

An example for a fed-state simulated intestinal fluid (FeSSIF) is: sodium taurocholate 15 mmol/L, lecithin 3.75 mmol/L, NaOH (pellets) 4.04 g, glacial acetic acid 8.65 g, NaCl 11.874 g, purified water to 1000 mL. The higher concentration of bile salt and lecithin compared to the FaSSIF reflects the situation in the small intestine in the fed state.

Super disintegrants

In the previous sections we have discussed how to increase drug dissolution and solubility. If one is to use a solid dosage form, however, dissolution steps are preceded by the disintegration of the dosage form itself, in most cases a tablet or capsule. If a fast onset of action is desired (such as in immediate-release dosage forms), it is necessary that the dosage form itself disintegrates quickly to allow for the drug to be dissolved. Fast disintegration of a tablet can be achieved by using effervescent tablet formulations.

Alternatively, fast-acting disintegrating agents can be used in the tablet formulation. The role of a disintegrating agent in a tablet formulation (or sometimes in a hard gelatin capsule) is to improve the dispersion of the dosage form in the fluids of the gastrointestinal tract. Dispersion usually occurs initially into granules from where dispersion into powder particles occurs. It is thus necessary to add a disintegrant before and after granulation, if an agglomeration step is used in the formulation of the tablet. Amongst the various excipients that can act as disintegrants the so-called 'super disintegrants' can be used if a fast disintegration, and thus a fast onset of drug action, is desired. Super disintegrants can be classified according to their chemical structure into starch, cellulose or poly(vinylpyrrolidone) derivatives. Examples include sodium starch glycolate, croscarmellose and cross-linked poly(vinylpyrrolidone). All of these have in common that they are cross-linked and water-insoluble. These properties lead to a strong and fast swelling behaviour of these polymers when in contact with water, which brings about a fast disintegration.

Summary

In this chapter we have discussed various ways of improving the solubility and dissolution rate of poorly water-soluble molecules. This is of great importance for many drugs today, and a sufficiently high dissolution rate and solubility are required to develop immediate-release drug delivery systems successfully. However, not only are the dissolution and solubility of a drug important for a rapid increase in the drug plasma concentration, but also how easily a drug can overcome biological barriers to be taken up into the body. Drug permeability is thus another important consideration, particularly in the development of immediate-release dosage forms. This will be discussed in the next chapter.

Self-assessment

After having read this chapter you should be able to:
- categorise methods to improve bioavailability of immediate-release dosage forms by increasing the solubility and dissolution rate of the drug
- explain the difference between a 'brick dust' and a 'grease ball' molecule
- discuss the pros and cons of using the following methods to improve drug solubility:
  - use of water-miscible solvents
  - salt formation
  - prodrug design
  - cyclodextrin complexation
- name examples of prodrugs used to increase solubility and bioavailability of drugs
- explain the general chemical structure of cyclodextrins
- classify lipids into their various classes on a physicochemical basis
- discuss the pros and cons of using lipid-based, water-free formulations to improve the bioavailability of drugs
- explain what SMEDDS and SEDDS are
- draw a schematic representation of the various forms of microemulsions
- compare the different approaches to improve drug solubility and dissolution rate on the particulate level

- explain why decreasing particle size leads to increased dissolution rate using the Noyes–Whitney equation
- give examples of medicines using nanosizing technology
- discuss possibilities of stabilising nanosized particles against aggregation
- discuss the pros and cons of using metastable polymorphic forms of drugs to improve their solubility
- define what crystalline polymorphs and solvates are
- discuss the pros and cons of improving drug solubility by using amorphous forms
- explain how the amorphous state can be generated
- explain how polymers can help to stabilise the amorphous form of a drug against crystallisation and give examples of polymers used in this context
- explain how to determine dissolution rate and solubility of a drug
- explain the terms FaSSIF and FeSSIF and discuss their use in dissolution studies
- explain the term super disintegrants and discuss their use in tablet dispersion.

Questions

1. **Indicate which of the following statements is/are correct (there may be more than one answer):**
a. Many modern drugs have low aqueous solubility.
b. The dissolution rate of a drug is a thermodynamic property.
c. Saturation solubility is the maximum solubility of the solute in the particular solvent at equilibrium conditions.
d. For a given drug the dissolution rate only depends on the type of solvent and temperature.
e. The bioavailability of a drug depends on its solubility and ability to cross biological membranes (permeability).

2. **Indicate which of the following statements is/are correct (there may be more than one answer):**
a. Approximately one-third of novel chemical entities coming out of drug discovery research have an aqueous solubility of less than $10\,\mu g/mL$.
b. Many poorly water-soluble drugs are lipophilic. Such drug molecules are sometimes termed 'brick dust molecules'.
c. Drug molecules that don't dissolve well in either water or oil are sometimes termed 'grease ball molecules'.
d. Options to improve solubility, dissolution rate and subsequent bioavailability of drugs at the molecular level include the use of salt forms of drugs, the use of prodrugs and the use of cyclodextrins to complex the drug.

e. Generally, solvents containing a hydroxyl group such as ethanol, propylene glycol, glycerol and poly(ethylene glycols) of varying molecular weights may be used as co-solvents to improve drug solubility.

3. **Indicate which of the following statements is/are correct (there may be more than one answer):**

a. Formulation of drugs as salts instead of the use of the drug in its acid or base form is the most commonly used method to improve aqueous solubility and dissolution rate.

b. To investigate the solubility increase upon salt formation, pH solubility curves should be determined.

c. As a general rule, for acidic drugs the pK_a of the counterion should be lower by 2 pH values or more compared to the pK_a of the drug.

d. As a general rule, for basic drugs, the pK_a of the counterion should be higher by 2 pH values or more compared to the pK_a of the drug.

e. Excessively high concentration of the counterion of the salt form in the biological environment of the drug may lead to a decrease in the solubility of the drug. This is known as the common-ion effect.

4. **Indicate which of the following statements is/are correct (there may be more than one answer):**

a. Prodrugs may be designed from existing drugs to improve drug solubility.

b. Prodrugs are compounds which have to undergo biotransformation after exhibiting a biological response, to avoid toxicity.

c. Prodrugs may be designed from existing drugs not only to improve drug solubility but also to increase drug stability.

d. Prodrugs may be designed from existing drugs not only to improve drug solubility but also to enable site-specific drug delivery.

e. A prodrug is not considered a novel chemical entity and therefore using prodrugs to improve a drug's solubility does not require a new approval process.

5. **Indicate which of the following statements is/are correct (there may be more than one answer):**

a. Cyclodextrins are spherical oligosaccharides.

b. Suitable poorly soluble drugs may be complexed within the cyclodextrin cavity to improve solubility and dissolution rate.

c. Several derivatives of these molecules have been synthesised, including a hydroxypropyl and a sulfobutylether derivative, to achieve a higher water solubility than the underivatised cyclodextrins.

d. The bioavailability increase of a drug in a drug–cyclodextrin complex can be calculated from the phase solubility curves.
e. At higher cyclodextrin concentrations the cyclodextrins or the drug–cyclodextrin complexes may associate to form larger complexes that can precipitate.

6. **Indicate which of the following statements is/are correct (there may be more than one answer):**
a. Colloids are particles in the micrometre size range.
b. Colloids may be formed by the dispersion of larger particles.
c. Colloids may be formed by associations of smaller molecules.
d. Submicron emulsions are examples of kinetically stabilised colloidal systems.
e. Macromolecule solutions, liposomal dispersions and microemulsions are examples of thermodynamically stable systems.

7. **Indicate which of the following statements is/are correct (there may be more than one answer):**
a. Various types of lipids are employed in pharmaceutical formulations, and they can be classified physicochemically according to their ability to interact with water.
b. Non-polar lipids are insoluble in water and do not form a monolayer on the water–air interface.
c. Class I polar lipids are insoluble and non-swelling lipids, for example lethicin.
d. Class II polar lipids are insoluble and swelling lipids, for example vegetable oils.
e. Class III polar lipids are soluble amphiphilic molecules (also termed surfactants).

8. **Indicate which of the following statements is/are correct (there may be more than one answer):**
a. SMEDDS can form submicron emulsions by being diluted with water in the gastrointestinal tract independent of the activity of bile salts and lecithin.
b. SEDDS can form microemulsions by being diluted with water in the gastrointestinal tract independent of the activity of bile salts and lecithin.
c. SEDDS and SMEDDS may improve absorption of drugs from the gastrointestinal tract and reduce food effects which may lead to unpredictable absorption.
d. SEDDS and SMEDDS often include surfactants such as Cremophor EL, Tween, Span, Labrafil, Labrasol, Gelucire and TPGS.
e. For thermodynamic reasons emulsions cannot be formulated to have droplet sizes small enough and stabilities high enough to allow intravenous administration.

9. **Indicate which of the following statements is/are correct (there may be more than one answer):**
a. Microemulsions are one-phase systems, more closely related to micellar solutions than to coarse emulsions.
b. A large energy input (e.g. homogenisation or ultrasonication) is necessary to form microemulsions when mixing the individual components.
c. Droplet-type microemulsions contain nanometre-sized oil or water droplets and are usually called water-in-oil or oil-in-water microemulsions, depending on the nature of the droplets.
d. Some combinations of oil, water, surfactant (usually a mixture of several surfactants) and co-solvent can form microemulsion systems spanning from very low to very high water concentrations in the phase diagram. These systems are called bicontinuous microemulsions.
e. Neoral is an example of a marketed self-microemulsifying ciclosporin formulation.

10. **Indicate which of the following statements is/are correct (there may be more than one answer):**
    The Noyes–Whitney equation links the dissolution rate of a drug to its saturation solubility and to the surface area of the drug particles: dissolution rate $= dX/dt = AD/h(C_s - X_t/V)$.
a. In the Noyes–Whitney equation A is the surface area of the dissolving particle.
b. In the Noyes–Whitney equation D is the diffusivity (diffusion constant) of the solvent molecules.
c. In the Noyes–Whitney equation h is the effective boundary layer thickness around the dissolving particle.
d. In the Noyes–Whitney equation C_s is the saturation solubility of the drug and X_t is the amount of drug dissolved at time t.
e. In the Noyes–Whitney equation V is the molecular volume of the solute molecules.

11. **Indicate which of the following statements is/are correct (there may be more than one answer):**
    In the case of very small particles (in the low nanometre size range) not only the dissolution rate but also the saturation solubility may be increased. For spherical particles the following equation can be applied: $S = S_0 \exp (2\gamma M/r\rho RT)$.
a. In the equation above S is the saturation solubility of the drug, and S_0 is the saturation solubility of an infinitively large particle of the drug (infinitively here means particles in the micrometre size range).
b. In the equation above γ is the surface tension of the particle.
c. In the equation above M is the molar concentration of the drug at S_0.
d. In the equation above r is the radius of the dissolution vessel.
e. In the equation above ρ is the density of the particle, R is the gas constant and T is the temperature.

12. **Indicate which of the following statements is/are correct (there may be more than one answer):**

a. Two techniques have been used to achieve nanosizing of drug particles: wet milling using bead mills and high-pressure homogenisation.

b. Particle sizes that can currently be achieved using nanosizing techniques range between 1 and 2 nm.

c. For very small particle sizes one of the main problems is to avoid aggregation.

d. Non-ionic and anionic surfactants may be added in the nanosizing process to avoid particle aggregation.

e. Polymeric stabilisers can also be used instead of, or in combination with, surfactants to avoid particle aggregation in a nanosizing process.

13. **Indicate which of the following statements is/are correct (there may be more than one answer):**

a. Polymorphs of a drug crystallise into different lattices. Their physical properties, such as their density and solubility, however, are identical.

b. Polymorphs of a drug are chemically identical.

c. Different polymorphic forms can be prepared by changing the crystallisation conditions.

d. Most modern drugs show polymorphism, frequently being able to crystallise in three or more forms.

e. Solvent molecules may form part of the crystalline structure when they are included in the lattice during the crystallisation process from the solvent. The general expression for such crystals, containing drug and solvent molecules, is hydrates.

14. **Indicate which of the following statements is/are correct (there may be more than one answer):**

a. The amorphous state is characterised by a lack of long- and short-range order between drug molecules.

b. Drugs in the amorphous state often have a significantly higher solubility and dissolution rate than their crystalline counterparts.

c. Co-melting the drug with a suitable polymer can be used to improve the physical stability of the amorphous system.

d. The glass transition temperature of an amorphous form should be lower than the storage temperature to achieve sufficient physical stability of the amorphous state against crystallisation.

e. Water acts as a potent stabiliser for amorphous drugs and dosage forms, increasing the glass transition temperature substantially even at low water concentrations.

15. **Indicate which of the following statements is/are correct (there may be more than one answer):**
a. The dissolution rate of a drug is independent of the conditions under which the test is performed.
b. Biorelevant dissolution media are used to predict the in vivo behaviour of the formulation mainly in the development process.
c. Super disintegrants are used to increase the solubility of a drug.
d. Super disintegrants can be classified according to their chemical structure into starch, cellulose or poly(vinylpyrrolidone) derivatives.
e. Super disintegrants are usually cross-linked and water-soluble.

Reference

United States Pharmacopeia and National Formulary (USP 29 – NF 24) (2006). Rockville, MD: United States Pharmacopeial Convention.

Further reading

Solubility and dissolution
Florence AT, Attwood D (2008) *FASTtrack: Physicochemical Principles of Pharmacy*. London: Pharmaceutical Press.
Sinko PJ (2005) *Martin's Physical Pharmacy and Pharmaceutical Sciences*, 5th edn. Philadelphia, PA: Lippincott, Williams and Wilkins.

Salt formation, prodrugs and cyclodextrins
Brewster ME, Loftsson T. Cyclodextrins as pharmaceutical solubilisers. *Adv Drug Deliv Rev* 59: 2007; 645–666.
Serajuddin ATM. Salt formation to improve drug solubility. *Adv Drug Deliv Rev* 59: 2007; 603–616.
Stella VJ et al. (2007) *Prodrugs: Challenges and Rewards*. Berlin: Springer.

Lipid-based formulations
Hauss DJ (2007) *Oral Lipid-Based Formulations. Enhancing the Bioavailability of Poorly Water-Soluble Drugs*. New York, New York: Informa Healthcare USA.
Kumar P, Mittal L (1999) *Handbook of Microemulsion Science and Technology*. New York: Marcel Dekker.
Sjoblom J (2006) *Emulsions and Emulsion Stability*, 2nd edn. Boca Raton: CRC Press.

Nanosizing, polymorphism and amorphous systems
Bernstein J (2002) *Polymorphism in Molecular Crystals*. Oxford: Oxford University Press.
Kaushal AD et al. Amorphous drug delivery systems: molecular aspects, design and performance. *Crit Rev Ther Drug Carrier Syst* 21: 2004; 133–193.
Kesisoglou F et al. Nanosizing – oral formulation development and biopharmaceutical evaluation. *Adv Drug Deliv Rev* 59: 2007; 631–644.

chapter 3

Immediate-release drug delivery systems II: increasing the permeability and absorption of drugs

Overview

In this chapter we will:

- describe the importance of drug permeability
- describe the Biopharmaceutics Classification System (BCS)
- describe how to predict low drug absorption
- discuss the barriers to oral drug absorption and formulation strategies employed to enhance drug absorption.

Introduction

We have already seen that both solubility and dissolution are key parameters in controlling drug delivery, particularly if a rapid onset of action is required from a solid dosage form. However, for a pharmacological action, absorption across epithelial barriers

KeyPoints

- For drug release solubility and dissolution are important.
- For absorption drug permeability is also a controlling factor.

or cell membranes is also generally required. Plasma membranes offer selective permeability depending on the nature of the drug substance. Therefore, for an effective action, the drug must not only be present in the molecular form but also have sufficient permeability to cross the plasma membrane of epithelial cells; therefore solubility, dissolution and permeability are key factors for drug delivery.

The Biopharmaceutics Classification System

The majority of immediate-release dosage forms are designed for oral delivery. Patient compliance for orally administered drugs is usually higher than for other

KeyPoints

- The BCS categorises drugs based on their solubility and permeability.
- The absorption of a drug can be predicted using the 'rule of five'.

dosage forms, administration is simple and convenient and the manufacturing process for oral dosage forms is fast and cost-effective compared to other dosage forms. For these systems it is clear that the drug must have sufficient solubility in the gastrointestinal tract and that after dissolution the drug is able to permeate through the gastrointestinal epithelium to be absorbed into the body. The BCS is a means of classifying drugs based on their solubility and permeability. It is shown in Figure 3.1.

Figure 3.1 The Biopharmaceutics Classification System (BCS).

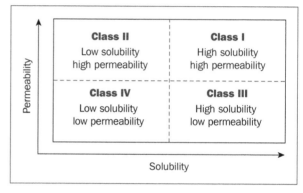

The two factors considered by the BCS are defined as follows:

1. Solubility: a drug substance is considered highly soluble if its highest dose strength is soluble in less than 250 mL water over a pH range of 1–7.5. This very practical definition reflects the fact that the liquid volume present in the gastrointestinal tract (in the fasted state) is approximately 250 mL and that the pH in the gastrointestinal tract varies from the stomach to the small intestine in the pH range used for the solubility determination. Solubility can be determined using pharmacopoeial methods.

2. Permeability: a drug substance is considered highly permeable if the absorption in humans is higher than 90% of an administered dose usually in comparison to an intravenously applied reference. However testing absorption in

Tips

1. The *permeability* (P) of drug molecules across a membrane is defined as:

$$P = (KD/\Delta h)$$

where K is the partition coefficient, D is the diffusion coefficient and Δh is the thickness of the membrane.

2. The *partition coefficient (oil/water)* (K) can be used as an indicator of the lipophilicity of a drug and is defined as:

$$K = C_{oil}/C_{water}$$

where K is the ratio of the concentration of unionised drug distributed between an organic (C_{oil}) and an aqueous (C_{water}) phase at equilibrium.

humans is costly and not always feasible at early stages of the developmental process. It is also possible to use in vitro methods to estimate permeability using either excised human or animal intestinal tissue or epithelial cell monolayers.

Predicting low drug absorption

In general permeability across the epithelial barrier and passive absorption of a drug are dependent on the drug concentration, the physicochemical characteristics of the drug and the area of absorptive tissue. Poor absorption can be predicted based on the physicochemical properties of a drug using the 'rule of five'.

Using this rule, poor absorption can be expected for drugs that have:

- more than *five* hydrogen bond donor groups (e.g. hydroxyl groups or amino groups)
- a molecular weight over *five* hundred
- a partition coefficient over *five*
- a sum of nitrogen and oxygen atoms in the molecules over 10 (2 times *five*) (the sum of nitrogen and oxygen atoms in the molecules is used as a measure of hydrogen bond donor and acceptor groups).

However this is only a guide; there is a range of drugs which are exceptions to this rule. In particular, active transport processes (rather than passive diffusion) for drug uptake are increasingly discovered for a range of drugs and the 'rule of five' may not apply in this case.

Tips

Models for drug absorption
In vitro
Cell culture models using the Caco-2 cell line are widely used as in vitro assays to predict absorption of drugs across the intestinal epithelial cell barrier. Caco-2 cells are an immortalised cell line of colonic tumour cells which have morphological and functional differentiation. They have distinct apical and basolateral domains, an apical brush border of microvilli and several brush border enzymes.
In vivo
These models generally involve monitoring appearance in the plasma as a function of time and can involve isolated intestinal segments.

Using the Biopharmaceutics Classification System

Using the BCS to consider both permeability and solubility, we can predict the possible rate-limiting factors for absorption of drugs and how these may be addressed.

Class I drugs

These drugs are well absorbed and their absorption rate is usually higher than their elimination rate, due to their high solubility and permeability. These drugs are especially suitable for the development of immediate-release dosage forms. If delayed-, sustained- or controlled-release dosage forms have to be prepared, addition of appropriate excipients and suitable formulation procedures are required.

Class II drugs

These drugs show limited bioavailability due to their poor solubility and/or poor dissolution rate. Improving the solubility or dissolution rate of these drugs is often possible by formulation approaches without having to change the nature (chemical structure) of the drug itself. Improving dissolution rate and solubility of this class of drugs and thus their delivery was discussed in Chapter 2.

Tips

Examples of drugs in the four classes of the BCS:
- Class I: paracetamol, diltiazem, metoprolol, propranolol
- Class II: carbamazepine, glibenclamide, ibuprofen, nifedipine
- Class III: aciclovir, captopril, cimetidine, neomycin B
- Class IV: hydrochlorothiazide, taxol.

Class III and IV drugs

These classes of drugs pose a bigger challenge because changing the permeability properties of the drug by formulation approaches is difficult. In such cases it is often the best option to optimise the chemical structure (and thus physicochemical properties) of the drug to improve absorption. This means a new chemical entity has to be synthesised, and this is usually time-consuming and costly. Increasingly in the pharmaceutical industry it is recognised that the properties of drug compounds should be optimised, not only to improve their pharmacological activity but also to improve their delivery properties (often now termed deliverability).

KeyPoints

- The amount of drug absorbed after oral administration is dictated by:
- the physicochemical characteristics of the drug (solubility and permeability)
- the conditions in the gastrointestinal tract (liquid volume and transit time).

The maximum absorbable dose

The amount of drug absorbed is a function of both drug permeability and drug concentration. Specifically for oral drug delivery systems the concept of the maximum absorbable dose (MAD) has been developed. The MAD is defined as:

$$MAD = SK_a V_i t_i$$

where:
- MAD is the maximum absorbable dose in mg
- S is the solubility of the drug in mg/mL at pH 6.5 (the average pH in the small intestine, the major absorption organ of the body)
- K_a is the intestinal absorption rate constant of the drug per minute
- V_i is the water volume in the small intestine (estimated as 250 mL)
- t_i is the transit time of the dosage forms in the small intestine (estimated as 270 minutes).

Like the 'rule of five', the MAD should only be regarded as a guide. However both are useful for ranking compounds in terms of potential bioavailability and to estimate target values for solubility in the drug development process. A problem in determining the MAD lies in predicting the solubility and permeability of the drug in in vivo conditions. The solubility of a drug can be highly dependent on the exact nature of the aqueous environment and is often different in buffer solutions compared to fluids of the gastrointestinal tract. Especially in the early stages of drug development, in vitro methods are used that may not fully reflect the situation in vivo.

Drug absorption

In the previous chapter we discussed various methods to increase solubility and dissolution rate for drugs to achieve a sufficiently high immediate release and to improve bioavailability. These approaches are useful for BCS class II drugs. However for class III and IV drugs, where permeability limits bioavailability, the approaches to improve bioavailability are more limited. In this section we will initially discuss the pathways of drug absorption as these are the basis for the approaches one can take to improve bioavailability for these classes of compounds. Again we are using the oral route as an example but the principles also hold true for other routes of administration.

> **KeyPoints**
> - The bioavailability of class II drugs can be improved by improving drug solubility.
> - To improve bioavailability of class III and IV drugs their permeability should be enhanced.

The human gastrointestinal tract

Orally administered drugs are mainly absorbed in the jejunum and ileum of the small intestine, but may also be absorbed in the buccal cavity, the stomach, the duodenum of the small intestine and the large intestine. The main reason for high absorption in the small intestine is the fact that the surface area available in this part of the gastrointestinal tract for drug absorption is very high compared to the other parts. The surface area available in the jejunum and ileum is approximately 60 m^2 in each of these two segments of the small intestine. In comparison, the surface areas available in the stomach and duodenum respectively are only 0.1 m^2, and in the large intestine 0.3 m^2. The large surface area in the small intestine can be explained by its anatomy. The intestinal mucosa consists of a single layer of columnar enterocytes and mucus-secreting goblet cells (these two cell types make up the epithelial cell layer), the lamina propria and a smooth-muscle cell layer of variable thickness,

> **KeyPoints**
> - Drug absorption in the gastrointestinal tract mainly occurs in the small intestine.
> - The jejunum and ileum have a large surface area for absorption due to the presence of villi and microvilli.
> - Drugs can be passively absorbed via diffusion through the cells (transcellular) or between the cells (paracellular). Alternatively drugs can cross the epithelium via active transport mechanisms.

consisting of 3–10 cell layers. The epithelium and the lamina propria protrude on their apical surface to form the so-called villi, which lead to a relative surface area increase in the small intestine by a factor of approximately 30. Moreover, the epithelial cells contain microvilli which further increase the surface area for absorption by a factor of approximately 600. On the surface of the epithelial cell layer is an aqueous, stagnant boundary layer (mucus layer). This hydrophilic layer, which varies in thickness from approximately 30 to 100 μm, is mainly composed of water containing negatively charged mucopolysaccharides (known as the glycocalyx), mucin (consisting of glycoproteins), enzymes and electrolytes. This hydrophilic layer may decrease the absorption of lipophilic drugs.

Tip

Whilst the passive diffusion process usually follows a first-order kinetics, active transport is saturable and often follows a Michaelis–Menten kinetics which in our context describes the dependence of the rate of absorption (V) when the concentration of the drug [D] present in the gastrointestinal tract is initially much larger than the concentration of the transporter T.

$$V = V_{max} [D]/(K_m + [D])$$

where:
- V is the observed absorption rate
- V_{max} is its limiting value at drug saturation (i.e. [D] $\gg$ K_m)
- K_m is the drug concentration when $V = V_{max}/2$.

Tip

ACE inhibitors inhibit the conversion of angiotensin I to angiotensin II. They are used in the treatment of heart failure and hypertension and for prophylaxis of cardiovascular events.

Drug absorption in the human gastrointestinal tract

Drug absorption in the small intestine can take place passively (by diffusion) either transcellularly (through the epithelial cells) or paracellularly (between the epithelial cells). The transcellular route of absorption is favoured by lipophilic drugs, whilst the paracellular route of passive transport is in principle favoured by hydrophilic drugs. In practice, however, it is often limited as the pores or gaps between the cells are very small (so-called tight junctions) and only comprise approximately 0.1% of the total surface area of the small intestine. In addition to passive transport, active, carrier-mediated transport mechanisms are increasingly discovered for a range of drugs (for example, antibiotics and angiotensin-converting enzyme (ACE) inhibitors), in which absorption is mediated by a transporter molecule carrying the drug across the cell membrane of the enterocytes or even through the whole cell.

Barriers to drug absorption

We have previously mentioned low solubility and slow dissolution rates as barriers to absorption (Chapter 2). But even if a drug is soluble in the gastrointestinal tract it faces many barriers for absorption. Whilst absorption of hydrophilic drugs is limited by the essentially lipophilic nature of the cell membrane of the epithelial cells and the limited availability of paracellular transport, lipophilic drugs may show limited absorption due to the presence of the aqueous stagnant boundary layer. Further, highly lipophilic drugs may not partition out of the cellular membrane and absorption could be hindered, therefore an optimum partition coefficient is usually observed for drug absorption.

Drug absorption from the gastrointestinal tract is also influenced by the residence time of the drug in the stomach, which can be quite variable and is influenced by the stomach content. Chemical and enzymatic degradation of the drug may occur in the stomach due to its low pH and the presence of digestive enzymes. Formulation solutions to this problem are discussed in Chapter 4.

Metabolism

Presystemic metabolism constitutes another barrier for drug absorption. In the case of oral administration we can differentiate between luminal and first-pass intestinal metabolism. Luminal metabolism is caused by the large number of digestive enzymes and other compounds responsible for drug degradation. Digestive enzymes that may degrade drug molecules include peptidases, proteases, lipases and esterases. The role of bile salts in luminal degradation has been mentioned in Chapter 2.

First-pass intestinal metabolism can occur by the brush border enzymes or inside the enterocytes. Brush border enzymes (phosphatases, peptidases and others) show the highest activity in the jejunum, followed by the ileum. Metabolism in the enterocytes includes the cytochrome P450 class, especially CYP3A4, which are phase I metabolising enzymes, but also a range of phase II metabolising enzymes. First-pass intestinal metabolism has to be differentiated from first-pass hepatic metabolism, which occurs after absorption of the drug and may be a major reason for low bioavailability after absorption of the drug from the small and large intestine (and to a variable extent from rectal absorption), due to the fact that after absorption the drug

KeyPoints

- Drug absorption of hydrophilic drugs can be hindered by the lipophilic nature of the epithelial cell membrane, whilst absorption of lipophilic drugs can be restricted by the aqueous, stagnant boundary layer.
- An optimum partition coefficient is often observed for absorption.
- Drug absorption can also be limited by enzyme degradation and metabolism of the drug.
- P-glycoprotein (PGP) pumps can also reduce absorption by effluxing the drug from cells.

Tips

Oral drug absorption is influenced by a range of factors, including:
- Gender: gastric acid secretion is lower and gastric emptying is slower in women than in men.
- Genetic profile: genetic differences in terms of enzyme expression influence drug bioavailability.
- Age: the pH profile in the gastrointestinal tract varies with age, and decreased enzyme activity is often found in the elderly.

Tip

During drug metabolism, the drug molecules are undergoing chemical biotransformation. These are commonly divided into phase I and phase II reactions. Phase I reactions increase the polarity of the drug molecules, for example by addition of polar groups (e.g. hydroxyl groups). In some cases phase I metabolism is sufficient for the metabolite to be excreted. Often, however, a second reaction takes place in which an endogenous polar molecule (e.g. an amino acid, glucuronic acid, sulfonates) is conjugated to the polar functional group, introduced in the phase I reaction. This process is known as a phase II reaction.

Tip

In general, if one chooses a delivery system other than oral or rectal forms, even though hepatic first-pass metabolism can be avoided, presystemic metabolism may still occur.

is transported to the liver by the portal vein before it reaches the systemic circulation.

Bacterial degradation

The gastrointestinal tract contains a range of microorganisms which aid digestion and support the immune system. The number of microorganisms increases from 10^2 colony-forming units (cfu) per gram of content in the stomach and duodenum, to 10^5 cfu in the jejunum, to 10^7 cfu in the ileum, to 10^{11} cfu in the large intestine. A consequence of this is that the likelihood of enzymatic degradation of the drug by enzymes of the bacterial flora also increases. Enzymes of the bacterial flora mainly include reductases, esterases, glycosidases and sulfatases.

P-glycoprotein drug efflux system

PGPs are membrane proteins that act as an effective drug efflux pump, transporting absorbed drug out of the epithelial cells of the small intestine (enterocytes) back into the gastrointestinal tract. They are usually co-localised with the enzyme cytochrome P450 3A4 (CYP3A4) at the apical surface of the cells and thus more efficient presystemic metabolism may be achieved as the drug is repeatedly absorbed back into the enterocytes and thus exposed for longer to the degrading enzymes. PGP is present in the enterocytes throughout the gastrointestinal tract but levels are higher in the colon than in the jejunum and in the stomach.

KeyPoints

- The absorption of drugs can be improved by:
  - formulating prodrugs with enhanced lipophilicity
  - using absorption enhancers to disrupt the epithelium barrier temporarily
  - blocking drug metabolism or efflux.

Strategies to overcome the barriers to drug absorption

Several of the strategies that a formulation scientist may use to improve absorption of drugs are similar strategies to the ones already discussed to improve solubility and dissolution rate (Chapter 2). These include the use of suitable prodrugs and of lipidic formulations. Other approaches are unique to increasing absorption and include the use of absorption enhancers and metabolism inhibitors.

Improving drug absorption by using prodrugs

Whilst we have seen that prodrug formation may lead to increased water solubility, it is also possible to create lipophilic prodrugs that may more easily overcome the absorption barriers of the gastrointestinal tract. A useful strategy is to convert carboxylic acid groups (or other polar groups such as phosphate groups) to lipophilic esters. Esterases in the body then convert the prodrug to its active form.

The ACE inhibitor enalapril is a prodrug showing better absorption than its active form enalaprilat, which was not suitable for oral application due to poor absorption (it was however suitable to be used as intravenous formulation due to its good water solubility). To produce enalapril one of the two carboxylic acid groups of enalaprilat is converted to an ethyl ester by an esterification reaction with ethanol. Enalapril is metabolised in vivo into the active form by the action of esterases.

Improving drug absorption by the use of absorption enhancers

Absorption enhancers are molecules that can be co-administered with the drug and that will lead to a temporary disruption of the barrier function of the epithelium. Absorption enhancement can be brought about by facilitating paracellular uptake and/or transcellular uptake or by disruption of the aqueous stagnant boundary layer. An example of a paracellular absorption enhancer is the chelating agent ethylenediaminetetraacetic acid (EDTA). This molecule binds calcium and magnesium which in turn leads to an opening of the tight junctions. Most transcellular absorption enhancers are surfactant-type molecules, such as the anionic surfactant sodium caprylate (sodium octanoate) and the non-ionic surfactants polyethoxylated castor oil (Cremophor EL) and polysorbate 80 (Tween 80). A major concern with the use of absorption enhancers is that, as they disrupt the barrier function of the epithelium, they may allow uptake of other compounds together with the drug and thus may have toxic effects.

Improving drug absorption by the use of metabolism inhibitors

As noted in the sections on metabolism and on P-glycoprotein drug efflux systems above, drugs can be metabolised by enzymes (e.g. CYP3A4) or their permeability limited by efflux mechanisms (PGP), resulting in low absorption. Molecules that inhibit these mechanisms can be co-administered with drugs to enhance absorption.

The protease inhibitor saquinavir is available in two formulations. Invirase (saquinavir mesylate) is formulated as a solid dosage form (capsules and tablets) and Fortovase (saquinavir) is a self-emulsifying drug delivery system formulation available in a soft gelatin capsule. When saquinavir is used as a single protease inhibitor in anti-human immunodeficiency virus (HIV) treatment, Fortovase is preferred as it has a higher bioavailability than

Invirase. However, Invirase may be used combined with ritonavir. As ritonavir is an inhibitor of CYP3A4, the co-administration of saquinavir with ritonavir substantially reduces metabolism of saquinavir and thus Invirase provides blood saquinavir levels at least equal to those of Fortovase.

When co-administered with ciclosporin, grapefruit juice can increase the bioavailability of this drug as grapefruit juice contains substances that selectively inhibit intestinal CYP3A4.

Summary

In Chapter 2 we discussed strategies to enhance dissolution and/ or solubility of drugs to increase their bioavailability and thus their usefulness as immediate-release drug delivery systems. In this chapter we have looked at methods to improve drug permeability, again with the aim of increasing drug bioavailability. The BCS shows that for class II drugs the former approaches are sensible and for class III drugs the latter approaches might be advantageous. For class IV drugs both types of approach may need to be employed. If dissolution, solubility and permeation are sufficiently high the drug can be developed into an oral immediate-release dosage form. In the next chapters we will see, however, that this is not always desired. In many cases, delayed-, sustained- and controlled-release dosage forms offer significant advantages over immediate-release dosage forms.

Self-assessment

After having read this chapter you should be able to:
- classify drugs according to the BCS
- predict absorption of drugs according to the 'rule of five'
- explain the term maximum absorbable dose
- discuss the absorption process of drugs, specifically for oral absorption
- discuss the role of cytochrome P450 and PGPs in oral drug absorption
- list the barriers for oral drug absorption
- explain how drug absorption can be improved using prodrugs
- discuss the pros and cons of using absorption enhancers and metabolism inhibitors to improve drug absorption.

Questions

Indicate if the following statements are true or false.
1. For an effective action, a drug must have sufficient permeability to cross the plasma membrane of epithelial cells.

2. The Biopharmaceutics Classification System (BCS) categorises drugs based on their solubility and bioavailability.

3. A drug substance is considered highly soluble according to the BCS if its highest dose strength is soluble in less than 50 mL of water over a pH range of 1–7.5.

4. The permeability (P) of drug molecules across a membrane is defined as: $P = KD/\Delta h$, where K is the partition coefficient, D is the diffusion coefficient and Δh is the thickness of the membrane.

5. The partition coefficient (oil/water) (K) can be used as an indicator of the lipophilicity of a drug and is defined as: $K = (C_{water}/C_{oil})$.

6. Poor absorption may be predicted based on the physicochemical properties of a drug, using the 'rule of five'; however, there are exceptions to this rule.

7. BCS class I drugs are well absorbed but their absorption rate is usually lower than their elimination rate.

8. BCS class II drugs show limited bioavailability due to their poor solubility and/or poor dissolution rate.

9. BCS class III drugs are commonly formulated as amorphous systems to increase drug solubility.

10. The maximum absorbable dose (MAD) is defined as: $MAD = SK_aV_it_i$, where S is the solubility of the drug in mg/mL at pH 6.5 (the average pH in the small intestine, the major absorption organ of the body), K_a is the intestinal absorption rate constant of the drug per minute, V_i is the water volume in the small intestine (estimated as 250 mL) and t_i is the transit time of the dosage forms in the small intestine (estimated as 270 minutes).

11. To improve bioavailability of BCS class III drugs their solubility should be enhanced.

12. For most drugs given orally drug absorption in the gastrointestinal tract mainly occurs in the stomach.

13. Drug absorption in the small intestine can only take place passively (by diffusion) either transcellularly (through the epithelial cells) or paracellularly (between the epithelial cells).

14. Oral drug absorption is influenced by a range of factors including gender, genetic profile and age.

15. Presystemic metabolism constitutes a barrier for drug absorption. In the case of oral administration one can differentiate between luminal and first-pass hepatic metabolism.

16. Cytochrome P450 (especially CYP3A4) are phase I metabolising enzymes present in enterocytes.

17. The number of microorganisms increases from 10^2 colony-forming units (cfu) per gram of content in the stomach and duodenum, to 10^5 cfu in the jejunum, to 10^7 cfu in the ileum to 10^{11} cfu in the large intestine.

18. P-glycoproteins (PGPs) are membrane proteins that act as an effective drug efflux pump, transporting absorbed drug out of the epithelial cells of the small intestine back into the gastrointestinal tract.

19. Absorption enhancers are molecules that can be co-administered with the drug and that will lead to a permanent disruption of the barrier function of the epithelium.

20. Ritonavir is an example of an inhibitor of CYP3A4. When ritonavir is co-adminstered with saquinavir, it substantially reduces the metabolism of saquinavir.

Further reading

General
Waterbeemd H *et al.* (eds) (2003) *Drug Bioavailability: Estimation of Solubility, Permeability, Absorption and Bioavailability.* Weinheim: Wiley-VCH.

Biopharmaceutics Classification System
Amidon GL *et al.* A theoretical basis for a biopharmaceutic drug classification: the correlation of in vitro drug product dissolution and in vivo bioavailability. *Pharm Res* 12: 1995; 413–420.

The 'rule of five'
Lipinski CA *et al.* Experimental and computational approaches to estimate solubility and permeability in drug discovery and development settings. *Adv Drug Deliv Rev* 23: 1997; 3–25.

Maximum absorbable dose
Johnson KC, Swindell AC. Guidance in the setting of drug particle size specification to minimize variability in absorption. *Pharm Res* 13: 1996; 1795–1798.

chapter 4

Delayed-release drug delivery systems

Overview

In this chapter we will:

- describe the ideal plasma concentration versus time profile of a delayed-release oral delivery system
- discuss the advantages of drug release in the small intestine
- describe how enteric coatings work and describe examples of enteric coatings
- discuss the advantages and disadvantages of colon-specific drug delivery
- describe strategies for colon-specific drug delivery.

Introduction

In Chapter 2 we discussed various methods of increasing the solubility and dissolution rate of drugs with poor water solubility. This is especially important if an immediate release of the drug is desired and if the bioavailability of the drug is depending on drug dissolution in the gastrointestinal tract, rather than being controlled by the permeation of the drug through the mucosal membranes to enter into the body (Chapter 3). In this chapter we will discuss methods of delaying the release of drugs from delivery systems in order to achieve drug release either in the small intestine or in the colon. Once the dosage form has reached the small intestine or the colon it is then desirable that the drug is released quickly and thus the resulting drug concentration versus time profiles resemble those of immediate-release dosage forms, but the time between administration of the drug and its release and thus appearance in the plasma is delayed. This has been shown schematically in Figure 1.3 in Chapter 1.

In most cases delayed release is achieved by coating the dosage form with

KeyPoints

- Oral drug delivery systems can be designed to delay drug release until the dosage form has reached the small intestine or the colon.
- Once these sites are reached, immediate release is required.
- This can be achieved using a range of polymeric coatings.

Tip

Polymer films are also used in the formulation of immediate-release dosage forms. The reasons for this include: facilitating swallowing of the dosage form, masking taste and odour, facilitating identification of the dosage form, enhancing the appearance of the dosage form, protecting the dosage form against environmental factors, such as light and moisture, protecting the dosage forms from breaking or abrasion during packaging or handling and improving the flow properties of pellets and granules. Such coats are dissolved quickly in the stomach and do not interfere with the release of the drug.

polymers that show no or only limited solubility in the parts of the gastrointestinal tract in which release is to be avoided but then release the drug quickly in the segments of the gastrointestinal tract where dissolution of the drug is desired.

Small intestine-specific delivery

KeyPoints

■ Enteric-coated dosage forms delay release until the small intestine is reached.
■ This can protect the stomach from the drug, protect the drug from degradation or provide targeted local delivery of the drug.

Enteric coatings are designed to prevent the release of the drug before the delivery systems reach the small intestine. The main reasons for enteric coating are:

1. The drug has to be protected from the acidic environment of the stomach against degradation.
2. The stomach has to be protected from the drug, which may lead to irritation when released in the stomach (i.e. to prevent gastric mucosal irritation).
3. The drug is supposed to act locally in the small intestine and a high drug concentration in this part of the gastrointestinal tract is desired.
4. Finally, if the drug is absorbed only in the small intestine, it may be beneficial to coat the dosage form enterically in order to achieve high drug concentration in the segment of the small intestine from which absorption occurs.

■ Examples of drugs that require protection from degradation include proton pump inhibitors of the azole type (omeprazole, pantoprazole) and antibiotics such as erythromycin and penicillin.
■ Examples of drugs that irritate the stomach include acetylsalicylic acid (aspirin) and other non-steroidal anti-inflammatory drugs such as naproxen.
■ Examples of drugs that are designed to act locally in the intestine include anthelmintics such as mebendazole and piperazine.

Mechanisms of enteric coatings

KeyPoints

■ Drug release in the small intestine can be achieved by pH-controlled release.
■ Polymers that are insoluble at stomach pH but dissolve at the higher pH conditions of the intestine are used.

The basic idea in enteric coating is to use polymers that are insoluble at low pH but soluble at a higher pH. The reason for this is that the pH in the stomach is usually 1.5–2 in the fasted state (but rising to approximately 4–5 in the fed state). In the small intestine, however, the pH is higher, usually between 6 (in the duodenum) and 6.5–7 (in the jejunum and ileum). Thus, if a polymer is used that is insoluble below pH 5 but soluble above pH 5, pH-triggered release in the small intestine can be achieved.

It is important that the dissolution of the polymer in the pH conditions of the stomach is as low as possible, as the residence time of the dosage form in the stomach is quite variable both between patients, but also for an individual patient depending on fasted or fed state. The residence time in the stomach also depends on the dosage form itself (size), with coated pellets leaving the stomach faster than intact tablets.

The pH-sensitive polymers used for enteric coating can be classified based on their chemical structure. Basically one can differentiate between cellulose derivatives, poly(vinyl) derivatives and poly(methacrylates). Often plasticisers have to be added to the polymer to obtain films that are forming readily in the coating process and that are flexible enough to avoid cracking. A crack in the polymer film will lead to dose dumping, which means the drug will be released too early, i.e. already in the stomach, and the aim of delayed release can no longer be achieved.

Tip

The mean residence time of a dosage form in the stomach can vary from less than 1 hour to many hours. For example, for enteric-coated tablets it has been found that the residence time in the stomach is on average less than 1 hour in the fasted state, 3–6 hours in the fed state and up to 10 hours if the patient is eating 'continuously', i.e. eating every 2.5 hours or less.

Tip

Plasticisers are additives that improve the pliability of a material. Plasticisers lower the glass transition of the polymer and make it more flexible and resistant to cracking. They can enhance spread of the coating over the tablets and granules. Examples include diethyl phthalate and glycerol.

The coating process

In most cases the polymer will be sprayed on to the solid dosage form as a solution or dispersion, using either fluid bed coaters or drum coaters. The coating fluid is sprayed on to the solid dosage forms, which may be tablets, pellets, granules, powders or microparticles. In some cases also capsules are coated. Hot air is introduced into the coater and leads to evaporation of the fluid and drying of the film coat. The polymer fluid should be applied on to the dosage form in small droplets and should have a low viscosity to ensure a uniform distribution on to the dosage form.

Polymer liquids can be applied in either aqueous dispersion or organic solution. If an organic solvent is used, the polymer will be molecularly dispersed in the solvent. If aqueous liquids are used, the polymer will be present in a particulate colloidal form (as a so-called latex dispersion). As the coating step and the drying step take place in the same machine, the entire coating process can be carried out without the risk of product being spread into the environment. When using organic solvents, the process machines have to be inert (to minimise the risk of explosion) and be used with a solvent recovery system (to minimise the environmental impact).

The film-forming process is different if the polymer is applied in an organic solvent or as a latex dispersion. If an aqueous dispersion is used, care must be taken that the temperature is high enough to allow the latex droplets to coalesce to form a uniform film. The lowest useful temperature of a specific film process is known as the minimum film-forming temperature. For some polymers it is necessary to add a plasticiser to the formulation to reduce the temperature necessary for film formation. The plasticiser also lowers the glass transition of the polymer and makes it more flexible and resistant to cracking. Plasticisers such as diethyl and dimethyl phthalate, glycerol, propylene glycol and triacetin are used. Other additives to the film-coating fluids include pigments, colorants, fillers, antitacking and antifoaming agents.

KeyPoint

- Polymers that can be used for enteric coating include cellulose derivatives such as cellulose acetate phthalate (CAP) and hypromellose phthalate, polyvinyl derivatives such as poly(vinyl acetate phthalate) (PVAP) and polymethacrylates.

Examples of polymers used for enteric coating

There are a range of pH-sensitive polymers that can be used for enteric coatings.

Cellulose acetate phthalate

CAP belongs to the group of cellulose derivatives. Approximately half the hydroxyl groups of the cellulose backbone are acetylated, and approximately a quarter are esterified, with half of the acid groups being phthalic acid (Figure 4.1a). Phthalic acid contains two carboxylic acid groups, so if phthalic acid is bound to the polymer backbone by one of its carboxylic acid groups, forming an ester with a hydroxyl group of the polymer, the second carboxylic acid group of phthalic acid remains free. This group can form salts in a weakly acidic, neutral and slightly alkaline, cation-containing environment. The resulting salt form of the polymer is soluble, the polymer coat of the solid dosage form can dissolve and the drug can be released from the dosage form.

CAP can be applied to solid-dosage forms by coating from either organic or aqueous solvent systems. The concentration of the polymer is usually in the range of 0.5–10.0% of the core weight of solid. Using CAP it is generally necessary to add a plasticiser to the polymer solution or dispersion. Plasticisers such as diethyl and dimethyl phthalate, glycerol, propylene glycol and triacetin can be used.

Hydroxypropyl methylcellulose acetate phthalate (HPMCAP: hypromellose phthalate)

HPMCAP also belongs to the group of cellulose derivatives (Figure 4.1b). It is a phthalic half ester of hydroxypropylmethylcellulose (HPMC). The pH value for rapid disintegration of HPMCAP can be controlled by varying the content of phthalic acid. Several qualities of this polymer are on the market which dissolve at either pH 5 (24%

Figure 4.1 Chemical structures of some polymers used for enteric coating. (a) Cellulose acetate phthalate (CAP); (b) hydroxypropyl methylcellulose acetate phthalate (HPMCAP); (c) methacrylic acid–methylmethacrylate copolymer (Eudragit L and Eudragit S).

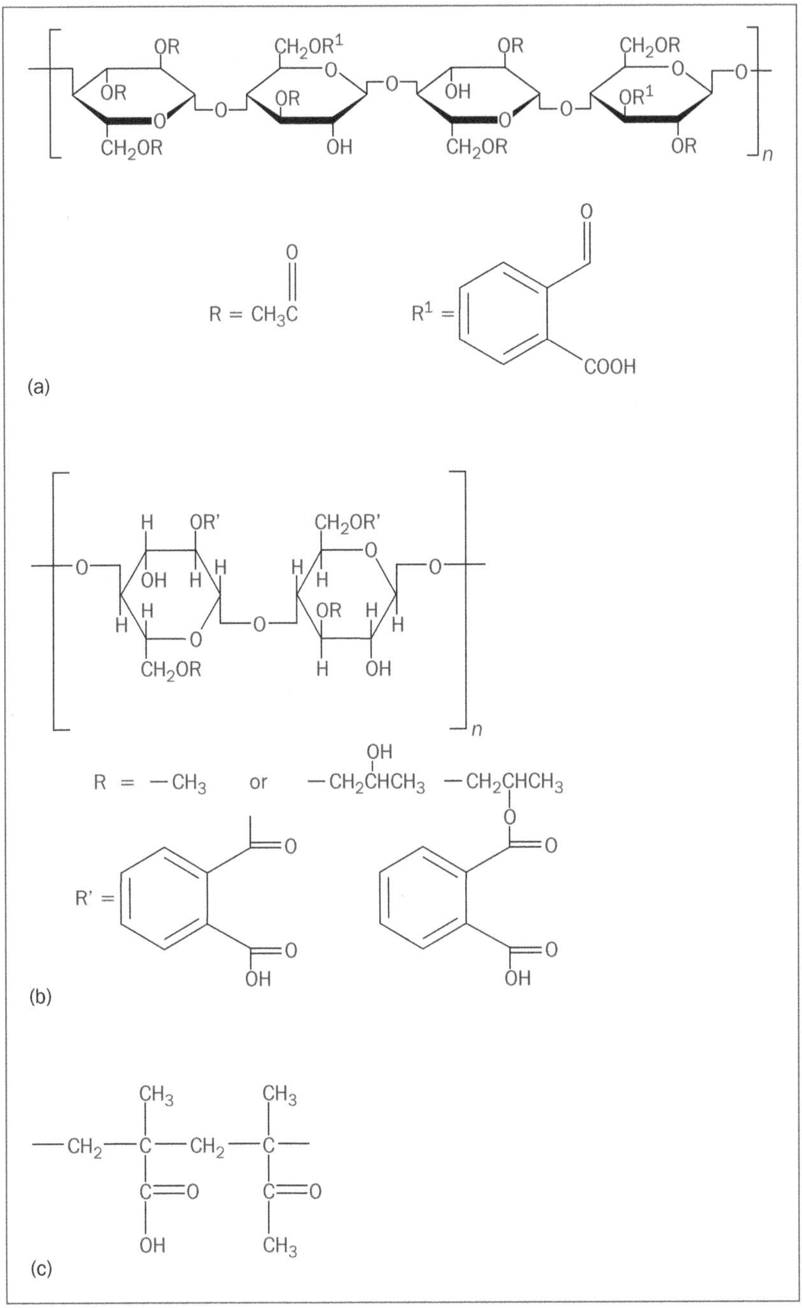

phthalyl content in the polymer) or pH 5.5 (31% phthalyl content in the polymer). Unlike CAP, HPMCAP is soluble in an ethanol/water (80:20) solvent mixture. It is also available as an aqueous dispersion. It is possible to use HPMCAP without the addition of a plasticiser, but to reduce the risk of cracks in the film, often plasticisers including triacetin, diethyl and dibutyl phthalate, acetylmonoglycerides and poly(ethylene glycol) 400 are added. Other polymers of the cellulose type that can be used for enteric coating include hydroxypropylmethylcellulose acetate succinate (HPMCAS) and cellulose acetate trimellitate (CAT), in which, instead of half esters of phthalic acid, half esters of succinic acid and partial esters of trimellitic acid are used to synthesise a pH-sensitive polymer.

Poly(vinyl acetate phthalate)

PVAP belongs to the group of polyvinyl derivatives. To synthesise PVAP, polyvinyl acetate is partially hydrolysed and the free hydroxyl groups are esterified with phthalic acid (the activated form of phthalic acid; phathalic anhydride is used for this reaction). This again leaves a free carboxylic acid group of the phthalyl group to render pH sensitivity of the polymer. PVAP is described as dissolving along the length of the duodenum. Organic (methanol, ethanol) and aqueous coating liquids are available for this polymer. Diethyl phthalate, polyethylene glycol 400, glyceryl triacetate and other plasticisers are commonly added to this polymer.

Polymethacrylates

These polymers are copolymerisation compounds of methylmethacrylate (which contains an ester function) and methacrylic acid (which contains a free carboxylic acid group). It is the free carboxylic acid group of the methacrylic acid parts of the polymer which makes the polymer pH sensitive. Like the free acid group of phthalic acid, succinic acid or trimellitic acid discussed above, this group remains unionised in acidic conditions and becomes ionised in neutral or weakly alkaline conditions. In fact, if the ratio of methylmethacrylate to methacrylic acid is 1:1, the polymer becomes soluble from around pH 5.5 to 6 onwards. A brand name for this polymer is Eudragit L (methacrylic acid:methylmethacrylate copolymer (1:1)). If the ratio of methylmethacrylate to methacrylic acid is 2:1, the polymer becomes soluble from around pH 6.5 onwards. A brand name for this polymer is Eudragit S (methacrylic acid:methylmethacrylate copolymer (1:2); Figure 4.1c). As with other enteric coating polymers, the polymer is available as organic solution (usually propanol–acetone mixtures are used), as aqueous dispersion or as a dry powder (which is then usually reconstituted in propanol–acetone mixtures). Dibutyl phthalate is used as plasticiser for these polymers.

Colon-specific drug delivery

The development of colon-specific drug delivery systems may be advantageous for the treatment of local and systemic diseases. Local diseases of the colon include colorectal cancer and Crohn's disease. However systemic adsorption after oral administration of colonic delivery systems has some advantages and disadvantages.

KeyPoints

- Site-specific delivery to the colon can avoid drug degradation in the low pH of the stomach and enzyme degradation in the small intestine.
- However drugs are subject to hepatic first-pass metabolism.

Advantages

1. For many drugs the pH conditions in the colon are more favourable than in the stomach. The proximal colon has a pH of approximately 6.4 and this value rises slightly to 6.6 in the transverse colon and to 7.0 in the distal colon.
2. The enzyme activity is much lower in the colon than in the small intestine.

Disadvantages

1. Absorption from the colon will lead to drug transport to the liver via the portal vein (if the drug is not absorbed directly into the lymphatic system), so that drugs subjected to hepatic first-pass metabolism will be significantly degraded before systemic circulation.
2. The concentration of microorganisms in the colon is very high and little is known about a possible presystemic drug metabolism by these microorganisms.

However, overall, the environment in the colon is less hostile for many drugs, particularly peptides and proteins, compared to that of the small intestine and the stomach.

Whilst colonic absorption has been demonstrated for a range of drugs, including diclofenac, metoprolol, nifedipine, theophylline and small-molecular-weight peptides, to improve drug absorption, co-administration of enzyme inhibitors, metabolism inhibitors and penetration enhancers may have to be used (Chapter 3). As for the small intestine, absorption is possible via the paracellular and the intercellular route. Active transport processes appear to be less common in the colon than in the small intestine.

Colon-specific delivery may be achieved by three different strategies: enzyme-triggered release, time-controlled release and pH-controlled release. Using enzyme-triggered release, both prodrug approaches and the use of polymers can be employed. Time-controlled and pH-controlled release can be achieved using suitable polymers.

KeyPoints

- Enzyme-triggered drug release exploits microorganisms present in the colon to release drugs by converting prodrugs to the parent drug or digesting polymer coatings on solid dosage forms.
- Polymer coatings that dissolve at pH 7 can be used to trigger release in the colon.
- Double coating of a dosage form with an outer enteric coat and an inner coat of a slow-release polymer can also promote release in the colon.

Enzyme-triggered release

Enzyme-triggered release is based on the idea of using the specific enzymatic activity of the microorganisms present in the colon either:

1. to convert prodrugs into the active form in the colon and thereby achieve uptake in this part of the gastrointestinal tract or
2. to use polymers that may be enzymatically degraded by the microorganisms and thereby lead to a release of the active compound in the colon.

Combination of the above-mentioned techniques: colon-targeted delivery system (CODES)

The CODES technique uses a combination of microbiological enzyme-triggered and pH-dependent mechanisms for site-specific drug release in the colon. The tablet consists of a core containing the drug together with the polymer lactulose and is coated twice, first with an acid-soluble polymer, e.g. Eudragit E, and then with a second enteric coating, e.g. Eudragit L (Figure 4.2). The enteric coating inhibits drug release from the tablet in the stomach and subsequently will quickly dissolve in the small intestine due to the increased pH. The inner acid-soluble coating then protects the drug from being released in the small intestine. However, gastrointestinal fluids can pass the acid-soluble coating layer and penetrate into the tablet core.

Figure 4.2 Principle of the CODES drug delivery system.

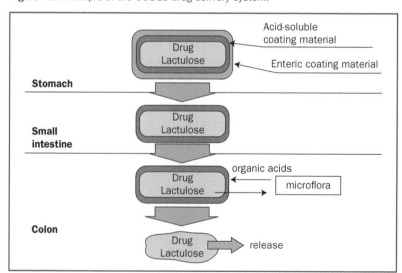

This leads to dissolution of the lactulose within the tablet. When the CODES then reaches the colon, lactulose leaches through the coating layer and is degraded by enterobacteria into organic acids. The reduction of the pH surrounding the tablet then results in dissolution of the polymer and subsequent drug release.

Prodrugs for enzyme-triggered release

An early example for the use of a prodrug in this context is the drug sulfasalazine. This drug was approved by the US Food and Drug Administration as early as 1950 and used in the treatment of Crohn's disease and inflammation of the colon. In the applied form the drug is inactive. The chemical structure of this drug (Figure 4.3a) shows that it contains an azo group (–N=N–). This group can be cleaved by bacterial diazoreductases into sulfapyridine and 5-aminosalicylic acid (Figure 4.3b and c). There is no diazoreductase activity in the upper parts of the gastrointestinal tract and limited absorption of the prodrug takes place in the small intestine. 5-Aminosalicylic acid clearly is an active drug, but whether sulfapyridine also has a beneficial effect is questionable. In fact it may be responsible for some side-effects of this drug. A further

Figure 4.3 Chemical structures of: (a) sulfasalazine; (b) sulfapyridine; (c) 5-aminosalicylic acid; (d) olsalazine.

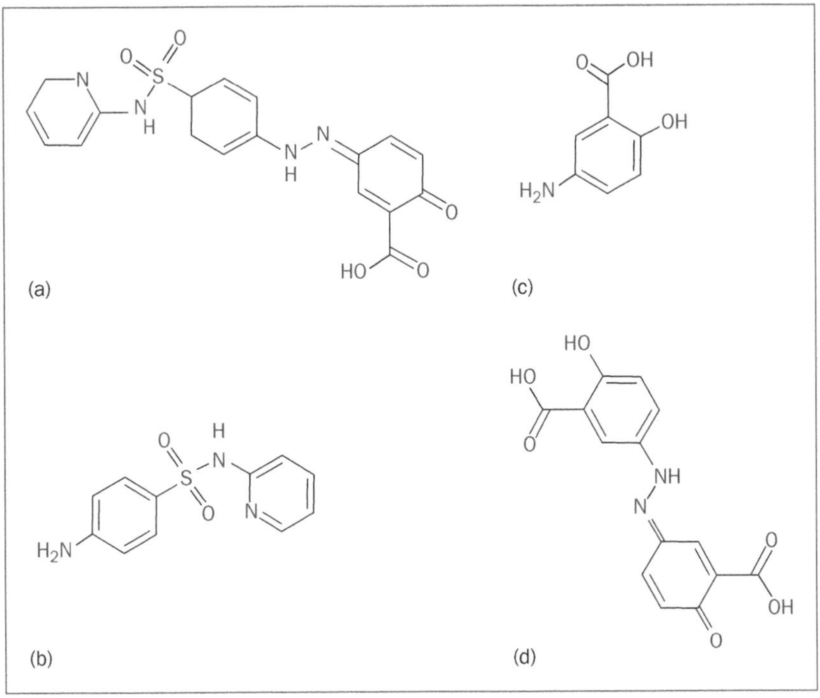

development of sulfasalazine is olsalazine which is a prodrug containing two molecules of 5-aminosalicylic acid linked by an azo bond (Figure 4.3d). Olsalazine is thus cleaved into two molecules of 5-aminosalicylic acid.

Polymers that can be considered for enzyme-triggered release include azo-group containing polymers coated on a solid dosage form (tablets, capsules or microparticles). There is, however, some concern about toxicity of the breakdown products of these polymers.

Natural and semisynthetic polysaccharides, including amylase, chitosan, cyclodextrins, guar gum, pectin, inulin and xylan, may also be used to achieve colon-specific delivery. These compounds are not digested in the upper parts of the gastrointestinal tract but are degraded by the microflora present in the colon. Whilst some of these compounds (amylose and pectin) can be used as film formers, if ethyl cellulose, for example, is added to stabilise the film, others have to be used as matrix materials in which the drug is embedded. A potential problem using polysaccharides is their relatively good water solubility. This can be significantly reduced by cross-linking the polysaccharide with glutaraldehyde.

Tip

As enzyme-triggered release relies on the presence of an intact and active microflora in the colon, care must be taken when antibiotics are administered as they may adversely affect the release of the drug. Also food might have an influence on the nature of the colon microflora.

pH-controlled release

We have seen earlier that poly(methacrylate) derivatives can be used as polymers for enteric coating. Depending on the concentration of free methacrylic acid groups, the polymers become soluble between pH 5.5 and 6.5 (Eudragit L and S). A similar concept has been used in Eudragit FS 30 D, which is an aqueous dispersion of a copolymer based on methylacrylate, methylmethacrylate and methacrylic acid. Unlike Eudragit L and S however, the ratio of the free carboxyl groups to the ester groups is approximately 1:10. This results in the polymer dissolving at a pH of 7. This pH is reached in the small intestine only in the distal parts of the ileum. If dissolution occurs here, the drug will pass into the colon through the ileocaecal junction. As discussed above, the pH initially drops to approximately 6 in the colon, so the dissolution of the polymer must be complete before the dosage form enters the colon.

Time-controlled release

Solely relying on the pH conditions in the small intestine to allow for a late dissolution in the ileum, but not in the upper parts of the small intestine, is not without risks. The pH in the upper parts of the small intestine may vary slightly and is not much below pH 7. Using Eudragit S (which dissolves above pH 6.5), for example,

Figure 4.4 Eudracol system for colonic release (see text for details). SR, slow-release.

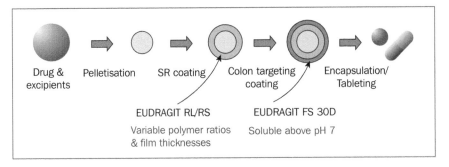

Drug & excipients → Pelletisation → SR coating → Colon targeting coating → Encapsulation/ Tableting

EUDRAGIT RL/RS
Variable polymer ratios & film thicknesses

EUDRAGIT FS 30D
Soluble above pH 7

Figure 4.5 Principle of the telescopic capsule.

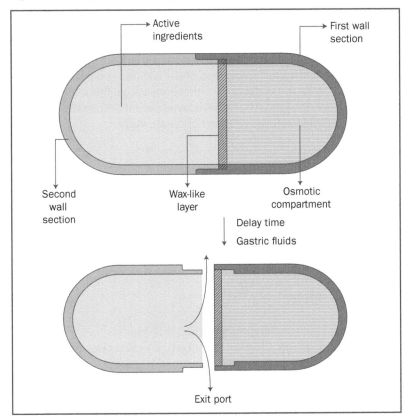

Active ingredients

First wall section

Second wall section

Wax-like layer

Osmotic compartment

Delay time

Gastric fluids

Exit port

has been shown to offer poor site-specific release. An approach combining delayed and slow release has been developed to give more reproducible colon-specific release. Essentially the drug formulation is coated twice. The inner coat is a slow-release polymer (Chapter 5) and the outer coat is an enteric coating polymer. The outer polymer prevents drug release in the stomach and the inner coat will retard release of the drug, so that most of the drug is in fact released in the colon. In this case drug release is not affected by pH, but depends on the nature and thickness of the inner coat.

An example of such an approach is the Eudracol system (Figure 4.4). Here the drug is initially incorporated into pellets. The pellets are then coated with a slow-release methacrylate derivative polymer (Eudragit RL/RS, see Chapter 5) and, in a second coating process, a Eudragit FS 30D coat is applied. The pellets are then filled into hard gelatin capsules or compressed to tablets.

Telescopic capsule as a delayed-delivery osmotic device

This capsule delivery device consists of two chambers, one containing the active ingredient and one containing an osmotic engine. Both compartments are arranged in a slidable, telescopic manner (Figure 4.5) and separated by a wax-like layer. During application, fluid imbibes the capsules, resulting in a volume increase of the osmotic chamber, while the volume of the reservoir with the drug stays constant. The continuous expansion of the osmotic compartment exerts pressure on the slidable capsule segments, pushing the first and second wall sections apart. After a delayed period of time the drug is then delivered through the exit port of the capsule.

Summary

Using polymeric coatings that can respond to changes in pH or enzymatic conditions supports delayed drug release from oral dosage forms until the small intestine or the colon is reached. However these systems delay but do not prolong the release of the drug. Methods of promoting sustained release of drugs will be discussed in Chapter 5.

Self-assessment

After having read this chapter you should be able to:
- draw an idealised plasma concentration versus time profile of a delayed-release oral dosage form
- discuss reasons for enteric coating of dosage forms
- briefly describe the coating process
- list examples of polymers used for enteric coating and give their general chemical structure
- describe the pH profile in the gastrointestinal tract
- discuss reasons for colon-specific drug delivery
- compare and contrast enzyme-triggered release, pH-controlled release and time-controlled release to achieve colon-specific drug delivery.

Questions

1. Indicate which of the following statements is/are not correct (there may be more than one answer):
a. Oral drug delivery systems can be designed to delay drug release until the dosage form has reached the small intestine or the colon.
b. Delayed release is in most cases achieved by coating the dosage form with poly(vinylpyrrolidone).
c. Enteric coatings may protect the stomach from irritations caused by the drug.
d. Enteric coatings may protect the drug against degradation from the acidic environment of the stomach.
e. Enteric coatings may provide targeted delivery of the drug to the liver and spleen.

2. Indicate which of the following statements is/are not correct (there may be more than one answer):
a. Examples of drugs that require protection from degradation in the stomach include omeprazole, pantoprazole, erythromycin and penicillin.
b. Examples of drugs that irritate the stomach include anthelmintics such as mebendazole.
c. Examples of drugs that are designed to act locally in the intestine include acetylsalicylic acid (aspirin) and other non-steroidal anti-inflammatory drugs such as naproxen.

3. Indicate which of the following statements is/are not correct (there may be more than one answer):
a. The basic idea in enteric coating is to use polymers that are insoluble at low pH and soluble at a higher pH.
b. The pH in the stomach is usually 3–4 in the fasted state (but rising to approximately 4–5 in the fed state).
c. In the small intestine the pH is higher, usually between 6 (in the duodenum) and 6.5–7 (in the jejunum and ileum).

4. Indicate which of the following statements is/are not correct (there may be more than one answer):
a. A plasticiser increases the glass transition of the polymer and makes it more flexible and resistant to cracking.
b. Plasticisers are additives to polymers that improve the pliability of the polymeric material.
c. Plasticiser can enhance spread of the coating over tablets and granules.

d. Examples of plasticisers used pharmaceutically include diethyl phthalate, glycerol and phenol.

5. **Indicate which of the following statements is/are not correct (there may be more than one answer):**
a. In most cases the polymer will be sprayed on to the solid dosage form as a solution or dispersion, using either fluid bed coaters or drum coaters.
b. Polymer liquids can be applied in either aqueous solutions or organic dispersions.
c. The polymer fluid should be applied on to the dosage form in small droplets and should have a high viscosity to ensure a uniform distribution on the dosage form.
d. The coating fluid is sprayed on to the solid dosage forms, which may be tablets, pellets, granules, powders or microparticles.
e. With aqueous polymer liquids care must be taken that the temperature is below the minimum film-forming temperature to allow the latex droplets to coalesce to form a uniform film.

6. **Indicate which of the following statements is/are not correct (there may be more than one answer):**
Polymers that can be used for enteric coating include
a. Cellulose acetate phthalate (CAP).
b. Hydroxypropyl methylcellulose acetate phthalate (HPMCAP).
c. Poly(vinyl chloride) (PVC).
d. Polymethacrylates (Eudragit L and Eudragit S).

7. **Indicate which of the following statements is/are not correct (there may be more than one answer):**
a. The proximal colon has a pH of approximately 6.4 and this value rises slightly to 6.6 in the transverse colon and 7.0 in the distal colon.
b. Absorption from the colon will avoid hepatic first-pass metabolism.
c. The concentration of microorganisms in the colon is very high and little is known about a possible presystemic drug metabolism by these microorganisms.
d. Colonic absorption has been demonstrated for a range of drugs, including diclofenac, metoprolol, nifedipine, theophylline and small-molecular-weight peptides.
e. Colon-specific delivery may be achieved by three different strategies: enzyme-triggered release, temperature-controlled release and pH-controlled release.

Further reading

Enteric-coated dosage forms

McGinity J, Felton LA (2008) *Aqueous Polymeric Coatings for Pharmaceutical Dosage Forms*, 3rd edn. Drugs and the Pharmaceutical Sciences 176. London: Informa Healthcare.

Colon-specific drug delivery systems

Lee VHL, Mukherjee SK (2006) Drug delivery: oral colon-specific. In: Swarbrick J (ed.) *Encyclopedia of Pharmaceutical Technology*. London: Informa Healthcare, pp. 1228–1241.

chapter 5
Sustained-release drug delivery systems

Overview

In this chapter we will:

- define the aim of developing sustained-release delivery systems
- describe the idealised plasma concentration versus time profile of:
  - repeated administration of an immediate-release oral dosage form
  - a sustained-release dosage form
- discuss the characteristics of drugs that make suitable candidates for sustained-release delivery systems
- explain the physicochemical basis of:
  - dissolution-based sustained-release delivery systems
  - gastroretentive sustained-release delivery systems
  - diffusion-based sustained-release delivery systems
- discuss methods to formulate these sustained-release drug delivery systems.

Introduction

In Chapters 2 and 3 we have discussed important issues for the development of immediate-release dosage forms. Immediate release is important to achieve a fast onset of action of the drug. To achieve this, the time to reach t_{max} in the plasma concentration versus time curve should be short. However, in many circumstances, this means that the duration of action of the drug will also be short. Maintaining the drug plasma concentration within the therapeutic range cannot easily be prolonged simply by increasing the dose, without reaching plasma concentrations that might be in the toxic range. In contrast, delayed-release dosage forms show a later onset of action (longer time to reach t_{max}) but they do not show a significantly increased duration of action. It is possible to prolong the time in which the drug plasma concentration is within the therapeutic range using repeated administration of an immediate dosage

KeyPoints

- Maintaining the drug plasma concentration within the therapeutic range can be achieved with repeated dosing of an immediate-release dosage form. However this leads to fluctuations in the drug plasma concentrations.
- Sustained release of drugs from delivery systems can provide prolonged drug release over an extended period, thereby extending the dosage intervals and reducing fluctuations in the drug plasma concentration profiles.

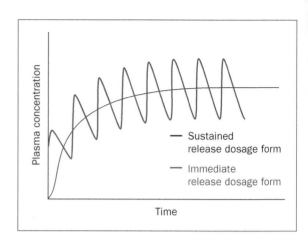

Figure 5.1 Idealised plasma concentration versus time profile of repeated administration of an immediate-release oral dosage form compared to a sustained-release oral dosage form.

form. However this leads to fluctuations (peaks and troughs) in the drug plasma concentration profile in the patient. This is shown in Figure 5.1.

It is not unusual for patients to forget to take a dose and even to attempt to compensate for this by taking twice the dose at the next administration time. This can lead to subtherapeutic levels on the one hand and unnecessary side-effects on the other. Therefore, for long-term treatment of many diseases it is beneficial for the patient if the dosing intervals can be prolonged, for example from two or three times a day (typical for immediate-release dosage forms) to once a day. This can increase the time the drug plasma concentration is within the therapeutic range, reduce adverse effects and increase patient compliance. An idealised plasma concentration versus time profile of a sustained-release oral dosage form is shown in Figure 5.1.

These possible advantages have led to the development of sustained-release dosage forms. We can define sustained-release dosage forms as drug delivery systems which provide the drug over an extended period of time. As for immediate and delayed release, we will discuss sustained-release forms using the example of oral dosage forms, as this route of administration is by far the most often used way to administer sustained-release dosage forms.

For a sustained-release system ideally we aim for constant drug plasma concentration levels over an extended time period. Therefore for oral delivery we require the rate of absorption of the drug from the gastrointestinal tract to be equal to the elimination rate (both by excretion and metabolism) of the drug. Whilst such a plasma concentration versus time profile can be achieved for intravenous infusion (and indeed from controlled-release dosage forms, which we will discuss in Chapter 6), it is not generally achieved for sustained-release dosage forms. This is because drug release from the dosage form may not be the rate-limiting step for absorption of the drug, and thus for its appearance in plasma.

Suitable drug candidates for sustained-release dosage forms

In addition to the formulation aspects of a sustained-release system, for a drug to be a suitable candidate for a sustained-release delivery system it needs to have a range of suitable properties.

KeyPoint

- Not all drugs are suitable candidates for sustained release and drug characteristics including dose, efficacy, solubility, stability, absorption and metabolism are important factors which must be considered.

Dose

For sustained release a drug should have a high potency and a low therapeutic dose. The typical weight of tablets or capsules to be easily administered orally is between 200 and 1000 mg. The dose administered in a sustained-release dosage form is usually two to three times that of an immediate-release dosage form of the same drug. For a drug that has a low pharmacological activity, this can mean that the dose becomes too large to be incorporated into a solid dosage form, especially taking into account that excipients have to be added to convert a drug into a solid dosage form.

Therapeutic range

A suitable drug candidate should have a large therapeutic range. If for some reason the total amount of the drug is released at once (for example, by poor coating or by chewing of the coated tablet), this may mean that toxic plasma levels can occur for drugs with a low therapeutic index.

Solubility

If a drug has a very low solubility, but still achieves sufficient plasma concentrations, it is usually not necessary to develop this drug further into a slow-release form. If the drug is absorbed during the whole gastrointestinal passage, absorption is controlled by the slow dissolution.

Stability in the gastrointestinal tract

Drugs for sustained release should not have a high degradation rate in the gastrointestinal tract. In the previous chapters we have discussed possible degradation of the drug by the low-pH environment in the stomach and enzymatic degradation in the gastrointestinal tract. Drugs that are subject to substantial degradation are unsuitable candidates for the development of sustained-release dosage forms. Although in total more drug is released from a sustained-release system compared with an immediate-release dosage form, at a given time lower concentrations of the drug are present in the gastrointestinal tract compared with immediate-release systems.

Absorption

A high absorption rate is advantageous for sustained-release drugs. Generally, absorption should be high for suitable drug candidates for the development of a sustained-release dosage form, so that the drug release rate is the rate-limiting step for the appearance of the drug in the body. As we have discussed previously, the transit time in the gastrointestinal tract is quite variable, mainly due to variations in the gastric residence time, whilst transport times in the small and large intestine are comparatively constant. It has been suggested that the minimal apparent absorption rate constant should not be lower than approximately 0.2/h to achieve complete absorption in the gastrointestinal tract, assuming a transit time in the adsorptive areas of the gastrointestinal tract of 8–12 h. Some drugs are taken up by active transport processes or only in a defined section of the gastrointestinal tract (adsorption window). These drugs are generally poor candidates to develop a slow-release dosage form as the time or regions for absorption are limited.

Presystemic metabolism

Presystemic metabolism (luminal and first-pass intestinal metabolism) of the drug after oral administration is of particular concern for slow-release dosage forms as the drug is present in low concentrations in the gastrointestinal tract. As metabolic processes involving enzymes are saturable, with enzymatic degradation often following a Michaelis–Menten kinetics, a low concentration of the drug will lead to a more complete enzymatic conversion.

Tips

A suitable drug candidate for the development of a sustained-release dosage form should have:
- a low therapeutic dose
- a large therapeutic window
- a high absorption rate
- a biological half-life between approximately 2 and 8 h.

A suitable drug candidate for the development of a sustained-release dosage form should not have:
- a low solubility
- a high rate of degradation in the gastrointestinal tract
- a narrow absorption window in the gastrointestinal tract
- a high rate of presystemic metabolism.

Half-life of the drug after absorption

Once the drug is released from the dosage form and absorbed into the body, it is subjected to metabolic and excretion processes that reduce the plasma concentration of the drug. These different processes are summarised as elimination. Elimination of the drug can be quantitatively described by the biological half-life of the drug $(t_{1/2})$, which is the time necessary to reduce the plasma concentration to half its original value. If a drug shows a short biological half-life, this means that the drug has to be administered frequently. These drugs strongly benefit from formulation as a sustained-release dosage form. However, care needs to be taken if the half-life becomes too short (shorter than 2 h), as in that case the dose necessary to be administered in a slow-release form may become too large to allow convenient oral administration in a solid dosage form. If the drug already shows a long half-life (longer than 8 h), there is rarely a need to develop slow-release dosage forms, as the biological effect of these drugs is already sustained.

Dissolution-based sustained-release dosage forms

As we have seen in Chapter 2, the Nernst–Brunner/Noyes–Whitney equation may be used to describe the dissolution rate of a drug as a function of its saturation solubility on the one hand and the surface area of the drug particles on the other hand.

$$\text{Dissolution rate} = \frac{dX}{dt} = \frac{AD}{h}\left(C_s - \frac{X_t}{V}\right)$$

where:

- A is the surface area of the particle
- D is the diffusivity (diffusion constant) of the molecule
- h is the effective boundary layer thickness around the dissolving particle
- C_s is the saturation solubility of the drug
- X_t is the amount of drug dissolved at time t
- V is the volume of solvent available for dissolution.

The dissolution process can be interpreted as a diffusion process of drug molecules through the effective boundary layer. This means that drug release is controlled by the diffusion of the drug molecule, once liberated from the drug particle, through the unstirred aqueous boundary layer.

In much the same way as decreasing particle size increases the drug dissolution rate, it is possible to lower the dissolution rate by increasing the drug particle size, by incorporating the drug in a slowly dissolving matrix (matrix dissolution dosage forms) or by coating the drug with a slowly dissolving film (encapsulated dissolution dosage forms).

Pellets can also be coated with a dissolving polymer coat of different thickness. For example, hydroxypropylmethylcellulose (HPMC) has been used to coat pellets in this way. The polymer forms an amorphous film, which is initially in the glassy state. Once the stomach fluids enter into the film, water lowers the glass transition temperature of the amorphous film and the polymer turns from the

KeyPoints

- The rate of drug release can be decreased by lowering the drug dissolution rate.
- This can be achieved by:
  - increasing the drug particle size
  - incorporating the drug into a slowly dissolving matrix
  - coating the drug with a slowly dissolving film.
- Compression of granules which have coatings that dissolve at different pH values can provide pulsatile release of the drug over the different regions of the gastrointestinal tract.

Tips

KeyPoints

glassy to the rubbery state. In this state the polymer starts to dissolve (but also diffusion of the drug through the polymer film occurs). The thicker the initial coat, the later the drug will be released.

Repeat action drug delivery systems

In order to increase the dissolution time it is also possible to formulate pulsatile (or repeat action) release systems. For example, it is possible to coat some granules with an enteric coat whilst others are not coated. If these granules are compressed into a tablet or filled into a hard gelatin capsule, dissolution of the drug will take place initially in the stomach (from the uncoated granules) and then again in the small intestine (from the enteric-coated granules). If several different enteric coating agents are used, dissolution at different pH values can be achieved, further increasing the time for drug release.

Gastroretentive drug delivery systems

Another approach to achieve prolonged release of a drug after oral administration is the use of gastroretentive systems. The idea here is to prolong the residence time of the dosage form in the stomach, called the gastric residence time. This is a useful approach, especially if drug absorption takes place in the stomach or the upper part of the small intestine (for example, in the duodenum), for local action of the drug in the stomach or for drugs with a narrow absorption window.

Several types of gastroretentive systems have been developed, which can be divided into:

- floating systems
- high-density systems
- expandable systems.

To understand these systems we need to have a look at the gastric motility in the fasted and fed state. In the fasted state, gastric motility can be divided into several phases, collectively called the interdigestive myoelectric motor complex (IMMC).

- Phase I (also called the basal state: approximately 45–60 min) is characterised by a relative absence of contractions.
- Phase II (also called the preburst state: approximately 30–45 min) is characterised by increasing frequency and strength of contractions.
- Phase III (also called the burst state: approximately 5–15 min) is characterised by strong contractions. Physiologically this phase serves to clear out the stomach of any undigested material and saliva and thus the contractions in this phase are also called 'housekeeper waves'.
- Phase IV (approximately 5 min) is a short period of no contractions after which the cycle starts again.

The situation is different if the patient is in the fed state as gastric emptying is significantly delayed by the presence of food in the stomach. Shortly after ingesting a typical meal the motor activity of the stomach starts to resemble that of phase II in the fasted state. This typically lasts for 3–4 h after a single meal. However, the exact time may differ depending mainly on the caloric value of the meal. The food is suspended into fine particles during this time. Particles smaller than 1 mm are emptied from the stomach through the pylorus into the duodenum in a zero-order fashion (approximately every 20 s). However, if the particles are larger than approximately 7–13 mm, they are retained in the stomach during this stage, and are emptied out into the duodenum during the next housekeeper wave. If the particles in the stomach become larger than approximately 5 cm in length and 3 cm in diameter, they become physically too large to empty into the duodenum even in a housekeeper wave.

These different situations in the gastric motility have consequences for the development of gastroretentive systems:

1. Gastroretentive systems should generally not be administered in the fasted state, as they could be emptied out of the stomach during the next housekeeper wave. The maximal length of time a normal sized delivery system can release drug in the stomach in the fasted state is approximately 2 h, but it is obvious that the release time will strongly depend on the phase during the IMMC at which the delivery system is administered.
2. A single-unit dosage form may be emptied out into the duodenum in an 'all or nothing' fashion. This makes drug retention times less predictable. Therefore it is generally advantageous to use multiple unit dosage forms, for example pellets, although several gastroretentive single-unit dosage forms have been developed successfully.
3. If gastric retention for longer times is desired, small gastroretentive systems rely on 'continuous eating' by the patient to avoid housekeeper waves. It is also possible physically to entrap the delivery system in the stomach, provided its dimensions are larger than approximately 5 cm in length and 3 cm in diameter.

KeyPoints

- Dosage forms with densities of less than approximately 1 g/cm^3 will float on gastric fluids. Sufficient fluid must be present in the stomach to support these systems.
- Hydrodynamically balanced systems use gel-forming hydrophilic polymers which swell and entrap air within the dosage form.
- Effervescent excipients such as bicarbonate or carbonate can be used to enhance buoyancy of delivery systems.

Gastroretentive drug delivery systems based on density differences to the gastric fluid

If the dosage form has a lower density than the gastric fluids, it will float on top of the stomach content, allowing for an increased time span to release the drug before the system is emptied out into the small intestine. The gastric fluid has a density of approximately 1 g/cm^3. If the density of the dosage form is lower than that, it will float on the gastric fluids. These systems require the presence of sufficient fluid in the stomach and the presence of food as discussed above. Several types of low-density single-unit dosage forms (tablets) and multiple-unit dosage forms (pellets) have been developed.

If the dosage form has a density of larger than approximately 2.5 g/cm^3, it will sink to the bottom of the stomach and pellets may be trapped in the folds of the gastric wall. Although the pellets are now closer to the pylorus (in the antrum of the stomach) it is possible that they withstand the strong peristaltic movements. To increase the density of the dosage forms barium sulfate, zinc oxide, titanium dioxide and other excipients may be used. However no marketed dosage form has been developed yet based on this principle.

Hydrodynamically balanced systems

In these systems the drug is encapsulated in a hard gelatin capsule together with a gel-forming hydrophilic polymer (Figure 5.2). HPMC is most often used for this purpose, but polymers such as hydroxyethylcellulose and sodium carboxymethylcellulose are also suitable. When the capsule shell disintegrates, the polymer forms a hydrated boundary layer. Through this layer drug can be released by diffusion. The hydrated boundary layer also entraps air in the inside, which results in an overall density of the system lower than that of the gastric fluid. Slowly the polymer erodes and the drug can be completely released. Additional to polymer and drug, lipophilic excipients such as vegetable oils may be added to the hydrodynamically balanced system to slow down water uptake and erosion and also to reduce the density of the system.

Examples of gastroretentive drug delivery systems based on density differences to the gastric fluid

- *Madopar.* Madopar is a marketed dosage form using a hydrodynamically balanced system. It contains levodopa and benseracid hydrochloride as active drugs. Levodopa has a short half-life and is also predominantly absorbed in the upper parts of the small intestine (absorption window in duodenum and

Figure 5.2 Schematic of a hydrodynamically balanced (HB) system.

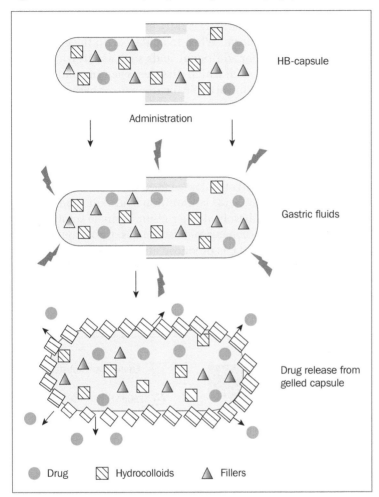

jejunum), and is thus a good drug candidate for this kind of drug delivery system.

- *Valrelease.* Valrelease tablets are another example of a gastroretentive drug delivery system based on density differences to the gastric fluid. The drug used in these tablets is the antidepressant diazepam. The drug is granulated with hydrogel-forming polymers which are then compressed into a tablet. After ingestion, the hydrogel formers take up water from the gastric juice and start forming a gel matrix around the core of the tablet. Drug release occurs in a controlled fashion via diffusion of the drug molecules through the gel layer. The density of the system stays below that of the gastric fluid and the tablet floats in the gastric content of the stomach.

- *Effervescent systems.* Another approach to achieve a low density for the gastroretentive dosage forms is to use effervescent substances in the formulation. Usually bicarbonate or carbonate is added to the dosage form. When in contact with the gastric fluid, the gastric acid (or additional acids such as tartaric acid, citric acid or ascorbic acid, which dissolve when in contact with the gastric fluid) converts the bicarbonate or carbonate into carbon dioxide (CO_2), which remains partially entrapped in the dosage form and provides the necessary buoyancy.

Example of the use of effervescent substances to achieve low density

- *Liquid Gaviscon* is a marketed dosage form based on this principle, containing antacids (aluminium hydroxide and calcium carbonate), which are dissolved in a sodium alginate solution that also contains bicarbonates and carbonates. Upon contact with the gastric fluids, CO_2 is produced and this turns the liquid formulation into a low-density gel (called a raft) which floats on the gastric fluid (Figure 5.3). This dosage form is used for local treatment (gastro-oesophageal reflux) and thus is a good candidate for this type of drug delivery system.

Figure 5.3 Schematic of a gastroretentive dosage form using effervescent substances in the formulation.

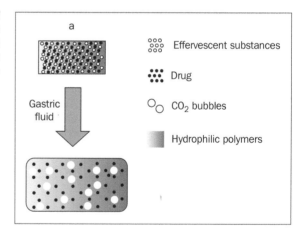

Swelling and expandable gastroretentive drug delivery systems

Conventional hydrogels swell slowly upon contact with water (or gastric fluid) due to their small pore size, which usually ranges in the nanometre and low-micrometre scale. However if the hydrogel has a pore size of more than 100 µm (so-called superporous hydrogels), swelling is much faster (and occurs in a matter of seconds to minutes) and may lead to a large increase in size. Swelling ratios of over 100 can be achieved (Figure 5.4). These swollen systems become too large to pass through the pylorus and thus may be retained in the stomach even after a housekeeper wave, provided they have a sufficiently high mechanical strength to withstand the peristaltic movements in the antrum of the stomach. Additionally, these systems also keep the stomach in an apparently fed state (as they fill the stomach to quite a degree), and thus they may delay the onset of a housekeeper wave.

A whole range of different expandable systems have been developed, but so far none of these systems has reached the market. However they have been used in clinical studies. Whilst superporous systems swell to a sufficient size to achieve gastric retention, expandable systems unfold to a size large enough to withstand gastric transit. Importantly, the systems initially need to be small enough to be swallowed easily, and they must not cause obstruction in the stomach. This is even more important if these dosage forms are taken on several occasions. Therefore expandable systems are made from biodegradable polymers containing the drug. They must not contain sharp edges that can lead to local damage in the stomach, yet they need to show

KeyPoints

- Using hydrogels with large pore sizes (superporous systems) allows the development of delivery systems that rapidly and strongly swell in size.
- Whilst superporous systems swell to a sufficient size to achieve gastric retention, expandable systems unfold to a size large enough to withstand gastric transit.
- The delivery system may become too large to pass through the pylorus, thereby promoting retention in the stomach.

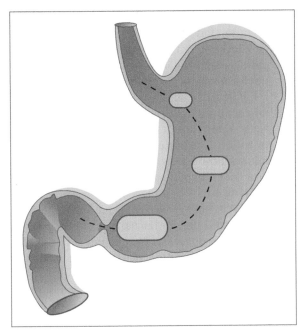

Figure 5.4 Schematic of the swelling and gastric transit of a superporous hydrogel.

Figure 5.5 Examples of expandable gastroretentive dosage forms.

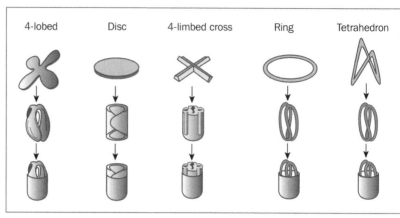

a certain rigidity to withstand the peristaltic conditions in the stomach. The systems are folded and usually put into a hard gelatin capsule. After the capsule disintegrates, the system expands/unfolds and the drug is then released by diffusion. In Figure 5.5 some examples of expandable gastroretentive dosage forms are shown.

KeyPoints

- Mucoadhesive polymers have been tried as a means of promoting retention by encouraging the dosage form to stick to the gastric wall.
- Magnetic dosage forms, held in place by an external magnet, have also been proposed.

Tip

Drugs that can delay gastric emptying (gastroparesis) include drugs for gastrointestinal conditions such as H_2-blockers, aluminium compounds, proton pump inhibitors, sucralfate and other drugs including anticholinergics, opiates, tricyclics and beta-blockers.

Other gastroretentive drug delivery systems

Besides the above-mentioned systems, a range of other approaches to achieve a longer gastric retention have been explored. Drugs can be co-administered with other drugs that delay gastric emptying. However, this approach is not favoured by clinicians.

It has also been suggested to use mucoadhesive polymers such as poly(acrylic acid), and chitosan to achieve gastric retention. The basic idea here is that the mucoadhesive polymer leads to the dosage form (usually pellets or microparticles) sticking on to the mucus of the gastric wall. Whilst the mucoadhesive approach is a sensible one for buccal and sublingual formulations (several buccal and sublingual tablets containing mucoadhesive excipients have been marketed), due to the rapid turnover of the mucus in the stomach, for gastroretentive systems this approach is not as straightforward.

Finally, magnetic materials may be added to the dosage form. These systems can then be held in place (for example in the stomach) by an external magnet, but this approach requires a precise positioning of the external magnet and is not likely to have a high patient compliance.

Diffusion-based sustained-release dosage forms

In the previous chapters of this book we have used the term diffusion on many occasions. In this section we discuss diffusion as a major principle to sustain drug release.

The process of diffusion

If we look at an oil-in-water emulsion under the microscope we can observe that the fine oil particles are undergoing irregular movements. They are performing a zig-zag motion. This motion is caused by the bombardment of the particles by molecules of the continuous phase (in our case the water molecules). Whilst we cannot see molecular motion of the water molecules themselves, we can see their effect on the dispersed oil droplets. The water molecules are colliding with each other and with the oil droplets because of the thermal energy they are subjected to. This phenomenon is known as random molecular motion.

Let us consider an individual water molecule colliding with other water molecules over a certain time t (Figure 5.6) due to random molecular motion.

Firstly, we have to determine an arbitrary x-axis. We can then determine the displacement of the particle in the x direction (Δx) after each time interval (Δt). As the displacement of the molecule is random, a large number of displacements will lead to a mean

> **KeyPoints**
>
> - Diffusion is the mass transport of individual molecules due to random molecular motion of the molecules along a concentration gradient.
> - Fick's first law of diffusion states that the amount of a drug in solution passing across a unit area is proportional to the concentration gradient across this unit area.

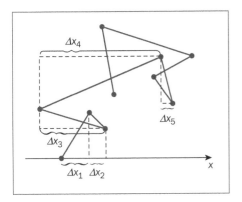

Figure 5.6 Path of a water molecule due to random molecular motion as a function of time.

displacement of zero (displacement can take place in x and $-x$ direction).

$$\overline{\Delta x} = (\Delta x_1 + \Delta x_2 + \Delta x_3 + \ldots \Delta x_n)/n = 0$$

However if we are using the square of the mean displacement the value will be unequal to zero:

$$\overline{\Delta x^2} = [(\Delta x_1)^2 + (\Delta x_2)^2 + (\Delta x_3)^2 + \ldots (\Delta x_n)^2]/n \neq 0$$

It can be shown that:

$$\overline{\Delta x^2} = 2\frac{kT}{f}\Delta t$$

where:

- k is the Boltzmann constant (1.381×10^{-23} J K^{-1})
- f is the coefficient of friction.

However as displacement of the water molecule may occur not only in the x direction (Δx) but also in the y and z directions, the total displacement $\overline{(\Delta s^2)}$ is therefore:

$$\overline{\Delta s^2} = \overline{\Delta x^2} + \overline{\Delta y^2} + \overline{\Delta z^2}$$

From this it follows that:

$$\overline{\Delta s^2} = 6\frac{kT}{f}\Delta t$$

With $f = 6\pi\eta r$, we can rewrite the above equation:

$$\overline{\Delta s^2} = 6\frac{kT}{6\pi\eta r}\Delta t$$

The expression ($kT/6\pi\eta r$) is also known as the diffusion coefficient or the diffusivity D (m^{2}s^{-1}). Therefore the above equation can be rewritten as:

$$\overline{\Delta s^2} = 6D\Delta t$$

This means that if a water molecule is at the centre of a hypothetical sphere at $t = 0$, after a certain time interval Δt, depending on the diffusivity of this molecule (in our example this is water) it will be somewhere on the surface of a sphere with the radius $r = \sqrt{\Delta s^2}$.

If we have a concentration gradient, that means if more molecules of a certain type are at one part of a system than at another, diffusion will occur along the concentration gradient of the system. We can therefore define diffusion as a mass transport of individual molecules due to random molecular motion of the molecules along a concentration gradient.

Fick's first law of diffusion states that the mass of a solute (for example, a drug in solution) passing across a unit area (this is known

Tip

The Boltzmann constant is the gas constant divided by the Avogadro constant. The coefficient of friction is the frictional force divided by the velocity of a particle in motion. In 1856 Stokes could show that for a sphere $f = 6\pi\eta r$, where η is the viscosity of the medium in which the particle moves and r is the radius of the particle.

as the flux J; units: kg m^{-2}s^{-1}) is proportional to the concentration difference across this unit area (dC/dx; units: kg m^{-4}). The proportionality constant is D (units: m^{2}s^{-1}).

$$J = -D(dC/dx)$$

This equation applies in steady-state conditions, which means dC/dx does not change with time (i.e. dC/dt = 0).

Reservoir systems

In Chapter 4 (dealing with delayed release) we have seen that coating a solid dosage form (e.g. tablets, granules, pellets, capsules) is a useful operation to delay the onset of drug release to the small intestine or the colon. We have discussed the properties a polymer needs in order to achieve this delayed release. It is also possible to use polymer coatings to achieve sustained release. For this purpose the polymer itself should not dissolve, but rather should allow the drug to diffuse through the polymer membrane to the outside, in the case of oral drug delivery, into the gastrointestinal tract. Therefore drug release should ideally be independent of the pH of the environment and should occur at the same rate throughout the gastrointestinal passage of the dosage form.

In a reservoir system, the drug is present in the core of the dosage form (termed the reservoir) and is surrounded by an inert polymer membrane (film). The release of the drug occurs by diffusion of drug molecules through the film. Therefore the nature of the film determines the drug release. We have seen that the flux of the drug molecules by diffusion can be described by Fick's first law of diffusion, i.e. $J = -D(dC/dx)$, as in most cases it is reasonable to assume that dC/dx does not change with time (dC/dt = 0).

Fick's second law of diffusion is the derivative of Fick's first law with respect to x. This law describes the diffusion of molecules in free solution and is used to describe the rate of change of the concentration of the diffusing molecules with time at a particular location.

To apply Fick's first law we have required that dC/dt = 0. We can thus rewrite Fick's second law in this particular case as:

$$D[d^2c/dx^2] = 0$$

As the diffusion coefficient D cannot be zero, it follows that $d^2C/dx^2 = 0$. As this is the second derivative of C with respect to x, the first derivative must be a constant: $dC/dx = $ constant. We therefore have a linear concentration gradient in a diffusion process following Fick's first law.

On the inside of the polymer membrane we have the drug reservoir. The concentration of drug in the reservoir is assumed to be constant. This is reasonable if there is an excess of drug in a solid form in the inside of the reservoir system, as only the drug in solution can diffuse though the membrane. The saturation concentration (C_s) of the drug in the reservoir is maintained by the dissolution of solid drug. For the process of drug diffusion out of the reservoir through the membrane and into the gastrointestinal tract it is therefore a prerequisite that water can diffuse through the film into the reservoir and dissolve a portion of the solid drug.

The concentration of the drug in the gastrointestinal tract can also be treated as constant because:

■ the concentration of the drug in the gastrointestinal tract is very low compared with the drug concentration in the reservoir (where we have saturation concentration)

■ released drug is absorbed into the body, further lowering the drug concentration in the gastrointestinal tract.

We can therefore assume so-called sink conditions, and the drug concentration in the drug reservoir and in the outside are practically constant over time, i.e. dC/dt is zero.

We can now replace the differential expression dC/dx by the expression:

$$(C_i - C_o)/h$$

where:

■ C_i is the effective drug concentration in the reservoir (this is the saturation concentration of the drug C_s)

■ C_o is the drug concentration outside the reservoir (this is the concentration of the drug in the gastrointestinal tract, and can often be treated as negligibly small)

■ h is the thickness of the polymer membrane.

However the drug will also partition into the membrane, as it will have a different solubility in the polymer membrane than in the reservoir of the fluids of the gastrointestinal tract. This will lead to a jump in the drug concentration from the reservoir (C_i) to the inner surface of the polymer film (C_{pi}) and from the outer surface of the polymer film (C_{po}) to the gastrointestinal tract (C_o). This is shown in Figure 5.7.

This situation can be accounted for by introducing the partition coefficient (K) of the drug into Fick's law: assuming that $K_i = C_{pi}C_i$ and $K_o = C_{po}/C_o$ are equal, we can replace K_i and K_o by a single

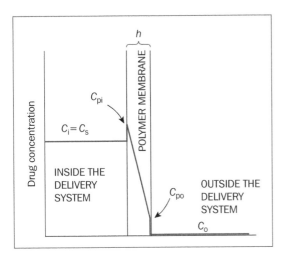

Figure 5.7 Schematic of the concentration gradient of a drug released from a reservoir system. In this example the drug solubility in the polymer membrane is higher than in the reservoir or in the gastrointestinal fluids. See text for details.

constant K and can now rewrite Fick's first law of diffusion for the case of membrane diffusion as:

$$J = -DK(C_i - C_o/h)$$

If we assume C_o to be practically zero, this equation is further simplified to:

$$J = -DK(C_i/h)$$

We now define the permeability (P) of the drug through the membrane as:

$$P = DK/h$$

and can rewrite Fick's first law as:

$$J = -PC_i$$

However a further complication has to be taken into account. We can assume that the polymer membrane will be situated between a stagnant aqueous diffusion layer, both in the inside and outside of the reservoir system, as shown in Figure 5.8.

We can again assume that the partition coefficient K of the drug is the same at the inside and outside of the polymer membrane, and that the concentration of the drug inside the reservoir system is constant ($C_i = C_s$) whilst it is practically zero on the outside (in the gastrointestinal tract). We then get the following relationship for the flux of the drug from the reservoir system:

$$J = \frac{D_m K D_a C_s}{h_m D_a + 2h_a D_m K}$$

Figure 5.8 Schematic of the concentration gradient of a drug released from a reservoir system. In this model the polymer membrane is situated between two stagnant aqueous diffusion layers. See text for details.

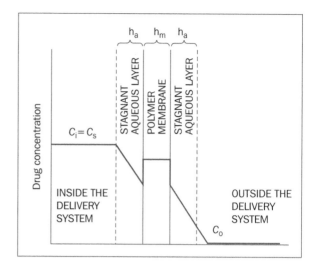

where:
- h_m is the thickness of the polymer membrane
- h_a is the thickness of the stagnant aqueous diffusion layer
- D_m is the diffusivity of the drug in the polymer membrane
- D_a is the diffusivity of the drug in the stagnant aqueous diffusion layer.

Depending on the properties of the diffusing drug, two cases can be considered. Either the membrane or the stagnant aqueous diffusion layer will control the drug release. Generally:
- Hydrophilic substances will diffuse slower through the polymer membrane than through the stagnant aqueous diffusion layer, and thus the membrane will control the overall release (membrane control).
- Hydrophobic drugs will diffuse slower through the stagnant aqueous diffusion layer than through the polymer membrane, and thus the stagnant aqueous solvent layer will control the overall release (solvent layer control).

In the case of membrane control the drug permeability through the polymer membrane (P_m) will be much smaller than permeability through the solvent layer (P_a):

$$P_m \ll P_a$$

From this it follows that we can neglect $2h_a D_m K$ from the above equation, which therefore simplifies to:

$$J = (D_m K C_s)/h_m$$

As D_m, K, C_s and h_m are all constants we can expect a zero-order drug release in the case of membrane control.

Similarly, in the case of solvent layer control, $P_m \gg P_a$ and hence we can neglect $h_m D_a$ in the equation $J = (D_m KD_a C_s)/(h_m D_a + 2 h_a D_m K)$, so that:

$$J = (D_a C_s)/2h_a$$

As in the case of membrane control, D_a, C_s and h_a are all constants and again we can expect a zero-order drug release in the case of solvent layer control.

Tip

$2h_a D_m K$ is present in the equation $J = (D_m KD_a C_s)/(h_m D_a + 2h_a D_m K)$ in the denominator as part of a sum, and can thus practically be neglected if it is very small compared to the other part of the sum, in this case: $h_m D_a$.

From the above we can conclude that, if both permeability and the drug concentration in the reservoir are constant, we should get a zero-order drug release. In reality this is often not strictly the case. For example, the polymer membrane may swell during exposure to the fluids in the gastrointestinal tract. This will affect the partition coefficient, K, and also the thickness of the membrane, h. Also, if the drug concentration in the reservoir becomes too low, i.e. if there is no more solid drug to dissolve, it can no longer be treated as a constant.

Furthermore, lag times and burst effects have to be considered. Immediately after preparation of a coated dosage form, the polymer will not contain any drug. If the dosage form is administered at this stage it will take some time for the drug to diffuse into the polymer coat from where it will be released. Therefore after administration, there will be a lag time until the drug will be released and can be absorbed into the body. On the other hand, in a coated delivery system that has been stored for a longer period of time, the drug might already have diffused into the polymer wall and this will lead to an initial burst release of drug shortly after administration. These effects are shown schematically in Figure 5.9.

However, in general, reservoir systems can lead to a near-zero-order release of drugs, which is advantageous for the release of the active molecule for a sustained period of time. These systems also have disadvantages though. Firstly, if the polymer is not dissolved or

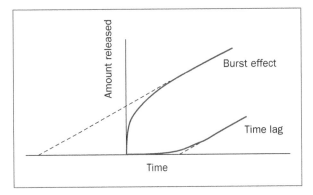

Figure 5.9 Schematic of drug release from a reservoir system showing a lag time in release and burst release. See text for details.

otherwise degraded, after passage through the gastrointestinal tract the dosage form may appear in the stool of the patient, who then might assume the drug has not been absorbed. If such dosage forms are used for administration routes other than oral delivery, they have to be removed from the body after the drug has been released. Also, if the polymer coat is faulty, so-called dose dumping may occur. This is a problem not only as the sustained-release character of the dosage form will be lost, but it may also lead to side-effects, as the minimal toxic concentration of the drug might be exceeded. This is possible, as the total amount of drug in a sustained-release dosage form is usually two to three times higher than in an immediate-release dosage form. The risk associated with dose dumping can be reduced if pellets or granules are coated instead of whole tablets or capsules. These coated particles can then either be filled in hard gelatin capsules or compressed into tablets. Care must be taken in the latter case to ensure that the compression process does not lead to damage of the polymer coats.

Polymers used in the development of reservoir systems

Two polymers commonly used as film formers in the development of reservoir systems are ethylcellulose and poly(ethylacrylate, methylmethacrylate, trimethylammoniummethacrylate chloride) copolymers (e.g. Eudragit RS and RL). It is possible to add a small quantity of a water-soluble polymer to the film former, to aid in drug release.

The chemical structure of poly(ethylacrylate, methylmethacrylate, trimethylammoniummethacrylate chloride) copolymers is shown in Figure 5.10. The presence of the permanently charged quaternary ammonium group gives the polymer the necessary polarity to allow water and drug diffusion after administration of the dosage form. Eudragit RL contains approximately double the amount of quaternary ammonium groups as Eudragit RS. Eudragit RS thus sustains drug release for longer than Eudragit RL.

Figure 5.10 Chemical structure of poly(ethylacrylate, methylmethacrylate, trimethylammoniummethacrylate chloride) copolymers.

$R_1 = H, CH_3$
$R_2 = CH_3, C_2H_5$

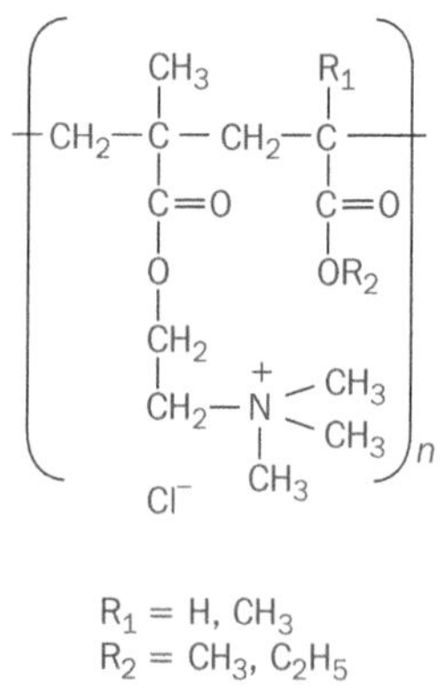

Matrix systems

Diffusion also governs the release from matrix systems. In these systems the drug is dispersed in a lipidic or more commonly a polymeric material which acts as the release matrix. Here we consider the case that the matrix is not soluble, such as in the case of an ethylcellulose or a poly(methacrylate) matrix, and the drug is partly dissolved in the matrix. The matrix can either be:

- homogeneous: the drug is partly dissolved and evenly distributed in the polymer matrix, or
- porous: here the matrix contains an additional soluble polymer which after administration dissolves quickly, leaving pores in the release matrix, or the matrix can simply be granular after formulation.

Homogeneous polymer matrix systems

In the case of a system containing the drug partially dissolved in a homogeneous polymer, it can be shown that drug release follows the equation:

$$Q = M/A = \sqrt{(D(2C_0 - C_s)C_s t)}$$

where:

- Q is the amount of drug released (M) per surface area (A) of the matrix system exposed to the release medium
- D is the diffusivity of the drug
- C_0 is the initial total drug concentration in the matrix system
- C_s is the solubility concentration of the drug in the matrix-forming polymer
- t is time.

If C_0 is very much larger than C_s, the above equation simplifies to:

$$Q = \sqrt{(D2C_0 C_s t)}$$

It can be seen from both equations (known as the Higuchi equations) that the release of the drug does not follow a zero-order kinetics but is a linear function of the square root of time, which means the release profile has the shape of a parabola as a function of time (Figure 5.11).

The reason for this release profile is explained schematically in Figure 5.12. Initially the drug is homogeneously dispersed throughout the matrix. When the dosage form is in contact with water, the water diffuses into the matrix and the drug diffuses out after water has entered the matrix (Figure 5.12a). After some time

> ## KeyPoints
>
> - In matrix systems the drug is dispersed in a lipidic or polymeric material that acts as a release matrix.
> - Release from matrix systems is controlled by diffusion and is related to the matrix type which can either be homogeneous or porous.
> - Drug release from matrix systems does not usually follow zero-order kinetics.
> - Drug release can be modelled using $Q/Q_\infty = kt^n$, where Q is the amount of drug released at time t and Q_∞ is the amount of drug released at infinite time. n is the release exponent.
> - Advantages of matrix systems over reservoir systems are that they are less expensive to produce and there is no risk of dose dumping.

Figure 5.11 Idealised release profile of a sustained-release matrix system.

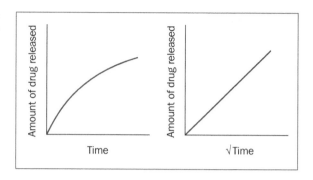

Figure 5.12 Drug release from a sustained-release matrix system. See text for details.

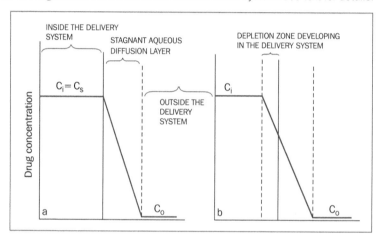

this will lead to the formation of a so-called depletion zone, which basically is a layer of drug-free matrix (Figure 5.12b). It follows that the remaining drug has to diffuse over a longer distance to be released. This is comparable to a reservoir system in which the membrane thickness increases (see above).

Porous polymer matrix system

In the case of a system containing the drug partially dissolved in a porous polymer, drug can leave the matrix by dissolving in the aqueous-filled pores of matrix. In this case, the solubility of the drug in the release medium becomes important, as well as the shape and volume of the pores in the matrix. The following form of the Higuchi equation has been derived to describe the release of the drug in this case:

$$Q = M/A = \sqrt{\left(D\frac{\varepsilon}{\tau}(2C_o - \varepsilon C_s)C_s t\right)}$$

where:

- ε is the tortuosity of the pores
- τ is the porosity of the delivery matrix.

As in the case of a homogeneous matrix, we can see that the drug release follows a square root of time function. Indeed, in both cases:

> Both ε and τ are dimensionless terms, which means that they have no units. τ is the total volume fraction of the matrix that can exist as channels or pores, and that can thus be filled with gastric fluid, and ε accounts for an increasing path length of diffusion due to bend pores and channels, compared to a straight channel.

$$Q = k\sqrt{t}$$

where k is a constant.

To be able to use the Higuchi equation to describe drug release from a matrix system, several assumptions have to be made:

- The polymer should not swell when exposed to the release medium.
- The diffusivity of the drug must remain constant during drug release.
- The polymer must not dissolve.

These prerequisites are not always fulfilled.

For example, the often-used matrix former HPMC swells and partially dissolves during drug release. To account for this behaviour, a power law has been introduced to describe drug release from matrix systems:

$$Q/Q_\infty = kt^n$$

where:

- Q is the amount of drug release at time t
- $Q\infty$ is the amount of drug released at infinite time
- n is the so-called release exponent.

If $n = 0.5$, the Higuchi equations are valid (remember: $\sqrt{t} = t^{0.5}$), and drug release can be assumed to be governed by fickian diffusion. On the other hand, if $n = 1$, drug is released in a zero-order fashion. This release kinetics is assumed to be due to release being controlled by polymer swelling. The amorphous polymer is initially in the glassy state, but with the diffusion of water into the matrix, the glass transition temperature of the polymer is lowered, as water acts as a plasticiser for the polymer. The polymer may then undergo a glass transition into the rubbery state, in which the molecular mobility of the polymer molecules increases, which leads to a higher diffusivity of the drug molecules and an increase in matrix volume. In this case, swelling of the polymer controls the release of the drug from the matrix system. In the field of polymer sciences this is known as case II transport. If the values for n are between 0.5 and 1, it is assumed that release of the drug from the matrix is governed by both fickian diffusion and case II transport.

An overall advantage of matrix systems over reservoir systems is that they are easier to produce and thus less expensive to

Tip

manufacture (no coating step is necessary in the dosage form development) and that dose dumping is unlikely to occur. Reservoir systems on the other hand allow for zero-order drug release which, as we have seen, is not usually achieved in matrix systems. An advantage of the swelling-controlled matrix systems over diffusion-controlled matrix systems is that burst release is unlikely to happen as the matrix has to swell first before a significant release of the drug occurs.

Polymers used in the development of matrix systems

Polymers used to develop matrix systems can be differentiated into hydrophobic and hydrophilic matrix formers. The hydrophobic matrix formers include poly(ethylene), poly(propylene) and ethylcellulose, and will usually lead to release that can be described by the Higuchi equations. On the other hand, more hydrophilic polymers, which include methylcellulose, hydroxypropylcellulose, HPMC, poly(ethylacrylate, methylmethacrylate) copolymers (e.g. Eudragit NE 40D, which has a ratio of 2:1 of ethylacrylate and methylmethacrylate units), poly(ethylacrylate, methylmethacrylate, trimethylammoniummethacrylate chloride) copolymers (e.g. Eudragit RS and RL), will often give rise to case II transport or a mixture of fickian diffusion and case II transport.

KeyPoints

- Bioerodible sustained-release systems release the drug due to erosion and/or degradation of the polymer matrix.
- Release depends on the geometry of the system.

Bioerodible sustained-release dosage forms

Bioerodible sustained-release dosage forms are matrix systems in which the drug is not primarily released by diffusion or dissolution, but in which the erosion and/or degradation of the polymer is the rate-limiting step for drug release.

The release mechanisms based on polymer erosion are complex and it has been difficult to describe the release process in simple equations, compared to reservoir or matrix systems in which the release is governed by diffusion. Moreover, as in the case of diffusion-controlled matrix systems, the release of drug from bioerodible sustained-release dosage forms depends on the geometry of the delivery system.

The following mathematical expression has been utilised to describe the drug release from these systems for simple geometries (slab, cylinder and sphere):

$$Q/Q_\infty = 1-(1-kt/C_0a))^n$$

where:

- Q is the amount of drug released at time t
- Q_∞ is the amount of drug released at infinite time
- C_0 is the initial drug concentration in the matrix system
- a is the half-height in the case of a slab geometry, or the radius in the case of a spherical or cylindrical geometry of the delivery system
- the exponent n has different values, depending on the system geometry:
- $n = 1$ for a slab
- $n = 2$ for a cylinder
- $n = 3$ for a spherical delivery system.

An advantage of bioerodible sustained drug delivery systems is that no 'ghost matrix' will be formed as in the case of matrix systems with insoluble and non-degrading polymers. However, it is more difficult to predict or control the release kinetics of these systems. Also, if polymer erosion is accompanied by polymer degradation, care needs to be taken to ensure that the degradation products are non-toxic.

Tips

Erosion of a polymer matrix can be defined as the loss of polymer mass from the matrix. This process may or may not be accompanied by polymer degradation.

Degradation of a polymer can be defined as a process in which the polymer chain is cleaved and which is thus accompanied by a reduction in the molecular weight of the polymer molecules. Degradation of the polymer may occur before significant weight loss of the polymer matrix (i.e. polymer erosion) occurs. This is the case for many poly(lactides) or copolymers of lactic and glycolic acid.

Polymers used in bioerodible sustained-release systems

Poly(lactides) or copolymers of lactic and glycolic acid are often used to formulate bioerodible drug delivery systems. Their chemical structure is shown in Figure 5.13.

Figure 5.13 Chemical structure of poly(lactic acid) and copolymers of lactic and glycolic acid.

Lactic acid

Poly(lactic acid)

X - Number of units of lactic acid
y - Number of units of glycolic acid

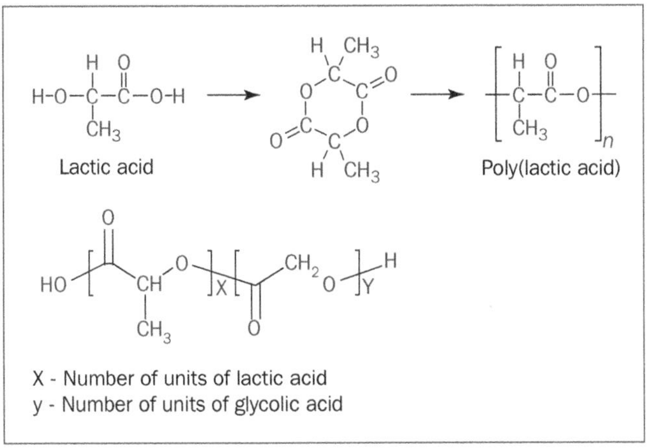

Summary

In this chapter we have reviewed the different release principles important in sustained drug delivery dosage forms. Whilst it is useful to differentiate the predominant processes including dissolution, diffusion, swelling and erosion, it should be remembered that often several of these principles are acting in parallel and influence the drug release from a sustained-release dosage form.

Self-assessment

After having read this chapter you should be able to:

- draw an idealised plasma concentration versus time profile of repeated administration of an immediate-release oral dosage form
- draw an idealised plasma concentration versus time profile of a sustained-release oral dosage form
- list and discuss the properties a drug should have to be a suitable candidate for the development of a sustained-release dosage form
- explain the physicochemical basis of dissolution-based sustained-release dosage forms
- explain what repeat action drug delivery systems are
- describe various methods to formulate gastroretentive drug delivery systems
- describe the various phases of the interdigestive myoelectric motor complex
- explain the principles of a hydrodynamically balanced system
- draw a schematic of the swelling and gastric transit of a superporous hydrogel
- explain the physicochemical basis of diffusion-based sustained-release dosage forms, using random molecular motion and Fick's law of diffusion
- describe drug release from a sustained-release reservoir system
- draw a schematic of the concentration gradient of a drug released from a reservoir system, using a model in which the polymer wall is found between two stagnant aqueous diffusion layers
- list polymers used in the development of reservoir systems
- compare and contrast matrix systems with reservoir systems
- describe drug release from a sustained-release matrix system
- explain drug release from a matrix system using the Higuchi equation
- list polymers used in the development of matrix systems
- explain the difference between bioerosion and biodegradation
- draw the chemical structure of poly(lactic acid) and copolymers of lactic and glycolic acid as bioerodible polymers.

Questions

1. **Indicate which of the following statements is/are correct (there may be more than one answer).**
a. The time in which the plasma concentration of the drug will be in the therapeutic range can be easily and safely prolonged simply by increasing the dose.
b. Delayed-release dosage forms show a later onset of action (longer time to reach t_{max}) and show a significantly increased duration of action compared to immediate-release dosage forms.
c. It is possible to prolong the time in which the drug plasma concentration is within the therapeutic range using repeated administration of an immediate dosage form. However this leads to fluctuations (peaks and troughs) in the drug plasma concentration profile in the patient.
d. It is not unusual for patients to forget to take a dose or even to attempt to compensate for this by taking twice the dose at the next administration time.
e. Especially in short-term treatment of diseases it is beneficial for the patient if the dosing intervals can be prolonged.

2. **Indicate which of the following statements is/are correct (there may be more than one answer).**
a. For sustained release a drug should require a low dose.
b. The typical weight of tablets or capsules to be easily administered orally is between 1000 and 2000 mg.
c. The dose administered in a sustained-release dosage form is usually two to three times that of an immediate-release dosage form of the same drug.
d. For a drug that has a low pharmacological activity the dose may become too large to be incorporated into a solid dosage form.

3. **Indicate which of the following statements is/are correct (there may be more than one answer).**
a. A suitable drug candidate for the development of a sustained-release dosage form should have a small therapeutic window.
b. A suitable drug candidate for the development of a sustained-release dosage form should not have too low solubility.
c. If a drug has a very low solubility, but still achieves sufficient plasma concentrations, it is usually not necessary to develop this drug further into a slow-release form.
d. A low absorption rate is advantageous for sustained-release drugs.

4. **Indicate which of the following statements is/are correct (there may be more than one answer).**
a. If a drug has a short biological half-life this means that the drug has to be administered frequently.
b. Drugs that have a long biological half-life (longer than 8 h) usually benefit from formulation as a sustained-release dosage form.
c. If the half-life of a drug is short (shorter than 2 h), the dose necessary to be administered in a slow-release form may become too large to allow convenient oral administration in a solid dosage form.

5. **Indicate which of the following statements is/are correct (there may be more than one answer).**
a. It is possible to decrease the dissolution rate of a drug by decreasing the drug particle size.
b. It is possible to slow down the release of a drug by incorporating the drug in a slowly dissolving matrix (matrix dissolution dosage forms).
c. It is possible to slow down the release of a drug by coating the drug with a slowly dissolving film (encapsulated dissolution dosage forms).
d. Pellets cannot be coated with a dissolving polymer coat of different coating thickness.

6. **Indicate which of the following statements is/are correct (there may be more than one answer).**
a. One approach to achieve prolonged release of a drug after oral administration is the use of gastroretentive systems.
b. The idea behind gastroretentive systems is to prolong the residence time of the dosage form in the small intestine, in particular in the jejunum.
c. Gastroretentive systems are a useful approach, especially if drug absorption takes place in the colon.
d. Gastroretentive systems are a useful approach for local action of the drug in the stomach, or for drugs with a narrow absorption window.
e. Several types of gastroretentive systems have been developed, including floating systems and expandable systems.

7. **Indicate which of the following statements is/are correct (there may be more than one answer).**
a. In the fasted state, gastric motility can be divided into several phases, collectively called the interdigestive myoelectric motor complex (IMMC).

b. In the fed state gastric emptying time is significantly increased by the presence of food in the stomach.

c. Gastroretentive systems should generally be administered in the fasted state.

d. A single-unit dosage form may be emptied out into the duodenum in an 'all or nothing' fashion.

e. If the particles in the stomach become larger than approximately 1 cm in diameter, they become physically too large to empty into the duodenum.

8. **Indicate which of the following statements is/are correct (there may be more than one answer).**

a. The gastric fluid has a density of approximately 2 g/cm^3.

b. In hydrodynamically balanced systems the drug is encapsulated in a hard gelatin capsule together with a gel-forming hydrophilic polymer.

c. Liquid Gaviscon is a marketed dosage form using a hydrodynamically balanced system.

d. Using hydrogels with large pore sizes (superporous systems) allows the development of delivery systems that rapidly and strongly swell in size.

9. **Indicate which of the following statements is/are correct (there may be more than one answer).**
    Fick's first law of diffusion may be written as: $J = -D(dC/dx)$.

a. In this equation J is mass of a solute (for example, a drug in solution) passing across a unit area.

b. In this equation the unit of J is: $\text{kg m}^{-2}\text{s}^{-1}$.

c. In this equation dC/dx is the concentration difference across this unit area.

d. This equation applies in steady-state conditions, which means dC/dx does not change with time (i.e. $dC/dt = 0$).

10. **Indicate which of the following statements is/are correct (there may be more than one answer).**

a. In reservoir systems, the drug is present in the core (reservoir) of the dosage form and is surrounded by an inert polymer film.

b. Drug release occurs by dissolution of the film.

c. Factors controlling drug release through the reservoir system film include the nature of the drug and the polymer film, the concentration gradient across the polymer film, the permeability of the drug across the polymer film and the polymer film thickness.

d. Reservoir systems usually show second-order drug release kinetics.

11. **Indicate which of the following statements is/are correct (there may be more than one answer).**
  a.   A polymer commonly used as film former in the development of reservoir systems is hydroxypropyl methylcellulose acetate phthalate (HPMCAP).
  b.   Polymers commonly used as film formers in the development of reservoir systems are Eudragit RS and RL.
  c.   Eudragit RL contains approximately half the amount of quaternary ammonium groups as Eudragit RS.
  d.   It is possible to add a small quantity of a water-soluble polymer to the film former to aid in drug release.

12. **Indicate which of the following statements is/are correct (there may be more than one answer).**
  a.   In matrix systems the drug is dispersed in a lipidic or polymeric material that acts as a release matrix.
  b.   Release from matrix systems is controlled by chemical degradation of the matrix.
  c.   The matrix type can either be homogeneous or porous.
  d.   Drug release can be modelled using $Q/Q_\infty = kt^n$, where Q is the amount of drug released at time t, Q_∞ is the amount of drug released at infinite time and n is the release exponent.
  e.   A disadvantage of matrix systems compared to reservoir systems is that matrix systems have a higher risk of dose dumping.

13. **Indicate which of the following statements is/are correct (there may be more than one answer).**
  In the case of a matrix system containing the drug partially dissolved in a homogeneous polymer, it can be shown that drug release follows the equation: $Q = M/A = \sqrt{(D(2C_0 - C_s)C_s t)}$. In this equation:
  a. Q is the amount of drug released (M) per surface area (A) of the matrix system exposed to the release medium.
  b. D is the molecular weight of the drug in daltons.
  c. C_0 is the final drug concentration in the matrix system 8 h after administration.
  d. C_s is the solubility concentration of the drug in the matrix-forming polymer.
  e. t is the temperature in Kelvin.

14. **Indicate which of the following statements is/are correct (there may be more than one answer).**
  a.   Bioerodible sustained-release systems release the drug due to erosion and/or degradation of the polymer matrix.
  b.   Release rates of bioerodible sustained-release systems are independent of the geometry of the drug delivery system.

c. Degradation of a polymer matrix is defined as the loss of polymer mass from the matrix.
d. Erosion of a polymer is defined as a process in which the polymer chain is cleaved and which is thus accompanied by a reduction in the molecular weight of the polymer molecules.
e. Degradation of the polymer may occur before significant weight loss of the polymer matrix occurs.

Further reading

Chien YW (1991) *Novel Drug Delivery Systems*. Boca Raton, FL: CRC Press.

Hadgraft J, Roberts MS (2003) *Modified-Release Drug Delivery Technology*. New York, NY: Marcel Dekker.

Mathiowitz E *et al.* (1999) *Bioadhesive Drug Delivery Systems: Fundamentals, Novel Approaches, and Development*. New York, NY: Marcel Dekker.

Senior J, Radomsky M (eds) (2000) *Sustained-Release Injectable Products*. Boca Raton, FL: CRC Press.

chapter 6

Controlled-release dosage forms

Overview

In this chapter we will:

- define the different aims of sustained and controlled release and identify the advantages of controlled release
- describe the ideal plasma concentration versus time profile of a controlled-release dosage form
- discuss the various mechanisms which can be used to give controlled drug release including the use of:
- polymer membrane permeation systems
- polymer matrix diffusion systems
- osmotic pressure-activated systems
- hydration and hydrolysis-activated systems
- feedback-regulated systems
- give examples of various controlled drug delivery systems that are on the market.

Introduction

In the previous chapter we have discussed methods to sustain drug release. The aim of these dosage forms is to slow down (prolong or retard) drug release in order to achieve a sustained drug plasma concentration within the drug's therapeutic window. In controlled-release delivery systems the aim is to attain control over the drug plasma concentration itself. In other words, to achieve reproducible drug release kinetics and get predictable and reproducible drug plasma concentrations. However, before we discuss the various controlled drug release dosage forms we will have a brief look at intravenous (IV) injections and infusions.

KeyPoints

- Drug infusions can give steady-state plasma concentration; however drug delivery via this route of administration is inconvenient.
- Controlled-release dosage forms are designed to give reproducible release kinetics and predictable drug plasma concentrations similar to infusions but without their limitations.

IV injections may be regarded as the ultimate immediate-release dosage form, in that the drug is already dissolved and is directly administered into the body. After an IV bolus injection usually a first-order decrease in drug plasma concentration is measured; the drug is immediately present in the plasma and only distribution and elimination processes influence the drug plasma concentration. Therefore

Tip

During a drug infusion, when the rate of drug infusion equals the rate of drug elimination the concentration in the body is balanced and a steady-state concentration is achieved. The steady-state concentration is the plateau concentration. It is the difference between the rate of infusion and rate of elimination that determines the amount of drug in the body at any time. Once the infusion has ended the plasma profile is similar to that of an IV bolus injection.

the plasma concentration is predictable, reproducible and controlled by the initial dose, the drug distribution and its elimination.

In the case of an infusion, after an initial increase in drug plasma concentration a steady-state concentration is reached depending on the infusion rate and elimination kinetics of the drug. In this situation the plasma concentration of the drug is constant. It is also predictable (provided the elimination kinetics of the drug is known), reproducible and can be controlled by changing the infusion kinetics. Once the infusion has been stopped, the plasma concentration of the drug decreases, usually in a first-order fashion. The differences in the plasma concentration versus time profiles of IV injection and infusion are shown in Figure 6.1.

Figure 6.1 Idealised plasma concentration versus time profiles of a drug after intravenous (IV) injection and infusion.

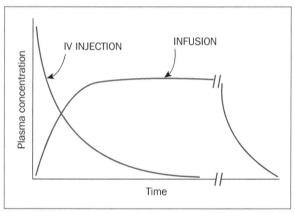

However, although drug infusions can provide controlled plasma levels, they have a range of disadvantages, including:

■ inconvenience for the patient
■ necessity for medical personnel to be involved in the administration
■ restriction to drug solutions and thus sufficient aqueous solubility of the drug
■ requirement for a sterile formulation.

The aim in developing controlled-release drug delivery systems is to achieve a similar plasma concentration versus time profile as would be achieved by administering drugs by infusion. Therefore for plasma concentration versus time curves of controlled drug delivery systems, 'the flatter the better' is a useful memory tool. However, not only has the plasma concentration profile to be flat, its steady-state level also has to be predictable.

The advantages of controlled-release dosage forms over conventional delivery systems include that the drug plasma concentration is at a predictable and desired level for a prolonged period of time. This avoids times of subtherapeutic drug concentrations and thus ineffective treatment, or too high drug concentrations that may lead to avoidable side-effects. This is shown schematically in Figure 6.2. Minimising dosing frequency will also enhance patient compliance. Drugs that benefit from delivery by controlled-release systems include those used for long-term treatments and/or if a constant plasma concentration is clinically relevant and beneficial. However we have discussed earlier that in some diseases variable plasma concentrations are actually more desirable than a constant plasma concentration.

Tip

An example of a drug where a constant plasma concentration is not desirable is insulin. Insulin is secreted by the pancreas in response to increased blood glucose levels. This stimulates cells to take up glucose from the blood and convert it to glycogen. At low insulin levels, glucose is not taken up and fat is used as an energy source. Therefore a variable insulin plasma concentration, which maps the plasma glucose levels, is the ideal situation.

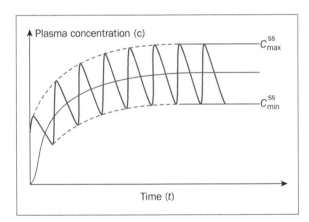

Figure 6.2 Idealised plasma concentration versus time curves of a drug delivered in several doses of an oral immediate-release dosage form and a controlled-release dosage form. C_{max}^{ss} and C_{min}^{ss} are the maximal and minimal steady-state drug concentrations after oral administration of the immediate-release dosage form respectively.

In previous chapters we have discussed immediate, delayed and sustained release, mainly focusing on oral dosage forms. This is justified not only because oral drug delivery is by far the most often used and most convenient route of administration, but also because for these types of delivery systems most research and development has been performed in the field of oral administration. This is not the case for controlled-release dosage forms. In this chapter we will therefore discuss the underlying principles and mechanisms in controlled drug release and review controlled-release dosage forms that have been developed for different routes of administration, including transdermal, ophthalmic, vaginal and parenteral delivery systems. It is beyond the scope of this book to discuss the specific anatomy of these delivery sites, and the reader is referred to Attwood and Florence (2008) for further information.

KeyPoints

- Drug release from polymer membrane permeation systems is controlled by diffusion.
- These systems comprise a drug reservoir enclosed within a polymeric coating.
- The polymer coating can be non-porous or microporous.
- Drug diffusion occurs through the polymer membrane or through pores in the membrane.
- Drug release is dependent on the drug concentration in the reservoir, the physicochemical properties of the drug and the properties of the polymer membrane.

Tip

Unlike conventional dosage forms which are characterised by a dose (for example, 100 mg of drug per tablet), controlled-release delivery systems are characterised by a release rate (for example, 20 µg of drug released per hour).

Polymer membrane permeation-controlled systems

The driving force for drug delivery in this class of controlled-release dosage forms is once again diffusion. Drug diffusion occurs through a polymer membrane or through pores in the polymer membrane. To achieve constant drug release the drug reservoir, which is encapsulated by the polymer wall, usually contains the drug in a solid form in a liquid or semi-solid dispersion medium. The drug concentration from which diffusion occurs is therefore constant (only drug in the saturated solution in the dispersion medium can diffuse), as long as excess drug is present in the solid form. Drug that diffuses out of the delivery system reduces the concentration of the drug in the dispersion medium but the concentration in the dispersion medium is maintained by drug dissolving into the medium from the solid drug particles. It follows that as long as drug is present in the solid form, a constant release rate and a zero-order kinetics profile may be achieved.

The polymer membranes used in these systems can be either:

- non-porous, in which case drug has to diffuse through the polymer, or
- microporous, in which case drug diffuses through the pores.

Figure 6.3 shows a schematic of these types of controlled-release drug delivery systems.

Figure 6.3 Schematic of polymer membrane permeation-controlled drug delivery system (a) with a non-porous polymer membrane and (b) with a porous polymer membrane.

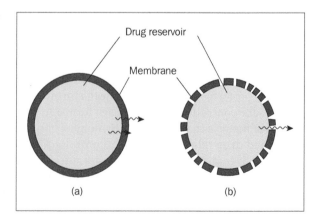

Drug release (Q/t) depends on the concentration of the diffusible drug inside the reservoir (C_r), diffusivity of the drug in the polymer membrane (D_m), diffusivity of the drug in the adjacent diffusion layer (D_d), the thickness of the polymer membrane (h_m), the thickness of the diffusion layer (h_d), the partition coefficient of the drug from the reservoir to the polymer membrane ($k_{m/r}$) and the partition coefficient of the drug from the polymer membrane to the aqueous diffusion layer ($k_{m/d}$). If the polymer membrane is porous, porosity of the membrane (ε) and tortuosity (τ) of the pores are also important factors determining the drug release rate.

All this appears very similar to our discussion on reservoir-type sustained-release dosage forms in Chapter 5. In fact the release principles are similar. However, the polymers used in controlled-release dosage forms are different (see below) and, for a suitable drug, the release kinetics determine the plasma concentration.

Examples of polymer membrane permeation-controlled drug delivery systems

Several dosage forms of this type have been successfully marketed for ocular, intrauterine, subcutaneous and transdermal applications.

Ocusert system

Ocusert is a controlled-release drug delivery system fabricated as an ocular insert. In this system (Figure 6.4) the drug (pilocarpine) is present in the reservoir as a drug–alginate complex. The polymer membrane is a microporous ethylene vinyl acetate copolymer. Tear fluid can penetrate through the membrane and dissolve the drug that can then diffuse through the membrane. Several systems have been designed with release rates of 20 or 40 µg pilocarpine/h. For the first few hours after administration, drug release rates are higher than 20 or 40 µg pilocarpine/h respectively, but within approximately 1 day after administration a constant release rate is achieved. The systems can be used for 4 or 7 days for the treatment of glaucoma. To facilitate localisation of the Ocusert system in the eye, the delivery system contains a white titanium dioxide ring.

Tip

For some controlled-release dosage forms the drug release kinetics may not be the rate-limiting step for absorption. This is the case for some transdermal controlled-release systems. We have used this strict definition here in order to highlight the principal differences between controlled- and sustained-release dosage forms.

KeyPoints

- Ocusert is an ocular insert which gives controlled release of pilocarpine. It has a drug–alginate complex reservoir and a microporous ethylene vinyl acetate copolymer membrane.
- Progestasert offers controlled release of progesterone. The drug is in a silicone matrix reservoir with a non-porous copolymer coating.
- Mirena is an intrauterine controlled-release system for levonorgestrel. Levonorgestrel is also available as a controlled-release subcutaneous implant (Norplant).
- Transdermal controlled-release systems (e.g. Transderm-Nitro) give controlled release across the skin. They utilise a porous ethylene vinyl actate copolymer membrane with the drug dispersed in a liquid silicone matrix.

Figure 6.4 Schematic of the Ocusert controlled drug delivery system.

13.4 mm

5.7 mm

74 μm

305 μm

Ethyl/vinyl acetate membrane

Pilocarpine reservoir

Titanium dioxide ring

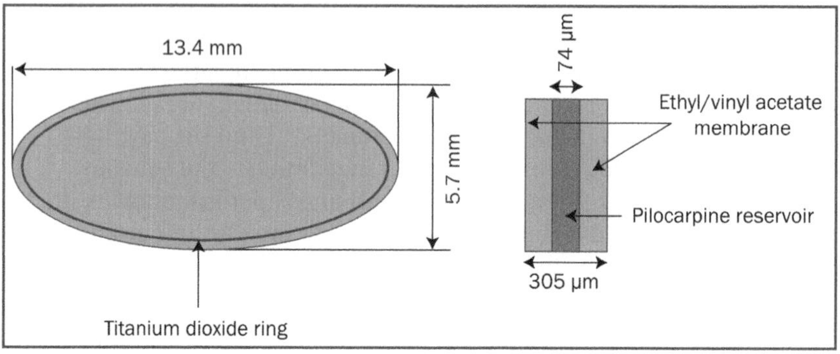

Progestasert system

Progestasert is a controlled-release intrauterine drug delivery system. In this system (Figure 6.5) the drug (progesterone) is present as a solid dispersion in a silicone matrix. The polymer membrane is a non-porous ethylene vinyl acetate copolymer. The system has been designed to release 65 μg progesterone/day and can be used for 1 year to achieve contraception.

Figure 6.5 Schematic of the Progestasert controlled drug delivery system.

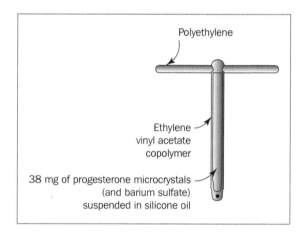

Polyethylene

Ethylene vinyl acetate copolymer

38 mg of progesterone microcrystals (and barium sulfate) suspended in silicone oil

Mirena system

Mirena is also a controlled-release intrauterine drug delivery system. In this system levonorgestrel is used as the drug. The system has been designed to release 20 μg levonorgestrel/day and can be used for up to 5 years to achieve contraception.

Tip

In contrast to ocular, intrauterine and transdermal controlled-release devices, implants cannot be easily removed from the body if one wants to end drug treatment.

Norplant system

Norplant is a controlled-release subcutaneous implant. In this system the drug (levonorgestrel) is present as a solid dispersion in a silicone matrix. The system has been designed to release 30 μg

Figure 6.6 Schematic of the Transderm-Nitro controlled drug delivery system.

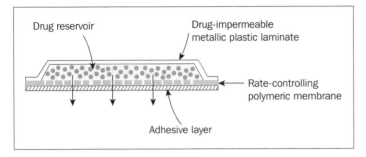

- Drug reservoir
- Drug-impermeable metallic plastic laminate
- Rate-controlling polymeric membrane
- Adhesive layer

levonorgestrel/day and has dimensions of 2.4 × 34 mm. The system can be used for up to 7 years to achieve contraception.

Transderm-Nitro system

Transderm-Nitro is a controlled-release transdermal drug delivery system. Controlled-release transdermal drug delivery systems are also often called transdermal therapeutic systems (TTS). In this system (Figure 6.6) the drug (nitroglycerine) is present as a solid dispersion in a liquid silicone matrix. The polymer membrane is a porous ethylene vinyl acetate copolymer. The system has been designed to release 500 µg nitroglycerine per cm² of the TTS per day for the treatment of angina.

Transdermal solid dispersions in a liquid silicone matrix

Similar TTS have been developed for transdermal delivery of:

- estradiol (Estraderm)
- fentanyl (Duragesic)
- testosterone (Androderm).

Polymer matrix diffusion-controlled systems

Similar to the previous class of controlled-release dosage forms, the driving force for drug delivery is again diffusion. However, by contrast, in this group of polymer matrix diffusion-controlled systems, drug is released through a polymer matrix, not through a polymer membrane. We have already discussed the release kinetics for such systems in Chapter 5 and the same principles

Tip

For controlled transdermal drug delivery the drugs should ideally penetrate easily though the stratum corneum of the skin. To be able to do this, the drugs should have a low molecular weight and be fairly lipophilic. As the stratum corneum of the skin is a very good barrier for absorption, this limits the number of suitable drugs for controlled release via this route.

KeyPoints

- Drug release is controlled by diffusion through a polymer matrix.
- The release profile of the drug is linear if plotted as a function of the square root of time.
- The choice of polymer–drug mixture will dictate whether controlled or sustained release is achieved.

apply here. Therefore, we do not see a zero-order release but usually a linear release of the drug as a function of the square root of time. By choosing the right polymer and drug, a controlled release can be achieved rather than the sustained release discussed in Chapter 5.

The drug is usually dispersed in the polymer matrix. This can be achieved by simply mixing the drug as solid particles into the polymer. In this case the polymer needs to be semisolid or liquid. However, polymers that are liquid or semisolid at room temperature or at body temperature will not lead to a controlled release of the drug but will at best lead to a sustained release. Therefore for controlled release, there are various options:

- After mixing the drug with the liquid or semisolid polymer, the polymer can be cross-linked in a second step after incorporation of the drug particles.
- It is also possible to heat a solid polymer above its softening point and incorporate the drug to the heated polymer. In this case the drug–polymer mixture simply needs to be cooled to room temperature to increase the viscosity or to solidify the system.
- If heat cannot be used, for example for stability reasons, it is also possible to dissolve the drug and the polymer in a common solvent and then to evaporate the solvent.

To give the delivery systems an appropriate form, the semisolid or heated polymer drug mixtures can be injection-moulded or extruded into the appropriate form. If a solvent evaporation technique is used this can take place in appropriately shaped moulds.

Compared to polymer membrane permeation-controlled systems no coating step is required and formulation is generally easier and more cost-effective. Also, no dose dumping can occur, for example through a faulty membrane. In fact, TTS of this type can be cut into smaller pieces, thus allowing individualisation of the release rate for the patient, without losing the controlled-release properties of the system. This is obviously not possible for polymer membrane permeation-controlled systems. On the other hand, as discussed above, the release rate is not usually following a zero-order kinetics, as in the case of polymer membrane permeation-controlled systems.

Tips

Polymer membrane systems
- Release controlled by drug diffusion through membrane
- Polymer coating can be non-porous or microporous
- Generally zero-order release profile
- Membrane integrity must be maintained

Polymer matrix systems
- Release controlled by drug diffusion through polymer matrix
- No coating required
- Generally linear release of the drug as a function of the square root of time
- Drug delivery systems can be subdivided, e.g. patches can be cut

Examples of polymer matrix diffusion-controlled drug delivery systems

Several dosage forms of this type have been successfully marketed mainly for transdermal and veterinary applications.

Nitro-Dur system

Nitro-Dur is a controlled-release transdermal drug delivery system. In this system the drug (nitroglycerine) is present as a solid dispersion in a hydrophilic polymer matrix. This drug–polymer matrix is then added on to an impermeable polyethylene cover strip on to which an additional occlusive aluminium foil is attached. Finally, an acrylic polymer tape is added in the form of an adhesive rim to place the delivery system on the skin (Figure 6.7). Drug release from this system is proportional to the area of the applied system and it releases 500 µg nitroglycerine per cm² of the TTS per day for the treatment of angina.

Nitro-Dur II and similar systems

Nitro-Dur II is a further development from the original Nitro-Dur TTS. The rate of drug release is again a linear function of the area of the applied system with a release rate of 500 µg nitroglycerine per cm² of the TTS per day for the treatment of angina. After 12 hours, the system has delivered approximately 6% of its original content of nitroglycerine. Again we can see that for controlled-release systems it is the release rate, not the drug dose, that is important. The Nitro-Dur II system contains nitroglycerine in an acrylic-based polymer adhesive with a cross-linking agent. The polymer thus serves a dual purpose as release matrix and as adhesive for skin application.

> ### Key Points
>
> - Nitro-Dur and Nitro-Dur II are matrix diffusion transdermal systems which give controlled-release rates of nitroglycerine proportional to the applied area of the system.
> - The Deponit system is also for controlled transdermal delivery of nitroglycerine. This system has several layers in the matrix, with decreasing drug concentrations. This leads to a zero-order release profile.
> - Zero-order release kinetics can also be achieved by coating a polymer matrix system with a polymer membrane.

Figure 6.7 Schematic of the Nitro-Dur controlled drug delivery system.

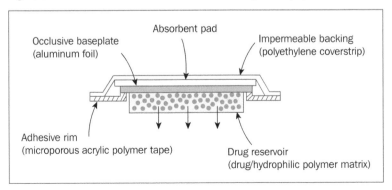

Acrylic-based polymer matrix systems

Other transdermal controlled drug delivery systems which use an acrylic-based polymer adhesive system with a cross-linking agent are:

- Climara, which delivers 17β-estradiol
- Habitrol, for 24-hour delivery of nicotine
- Minitran, for 24-hour delivery of nitroglycerine
- Nicotrol, for 24-hour delivery of nicotine
- Testoderm, for 24-hour delivery of testosterone.

Deponit system

In this polymer matrix diffusion-controlled transdermal drug delivery system the active agent is again nitroglycerine. In contrast to the previous systems the drug concentration in the matrix is not uniform, but different drug concentrations are present in several layers of the matrix. The layer closest to the adhesive layer has the lowest drug concentration and the matrix layer closest to the impermeable backing foil has the highest drug concentration (Figure 6.8). To achieve effective different drug concentrations of diffusible drug the drug has to be dissolved in the polymer matrix. This arrangement leads to a zero-order release profile at a release rate of 500 µg of nitroglycerine per day.

Figure 6.8 Schematic of the deponit controlled drug delivery system.

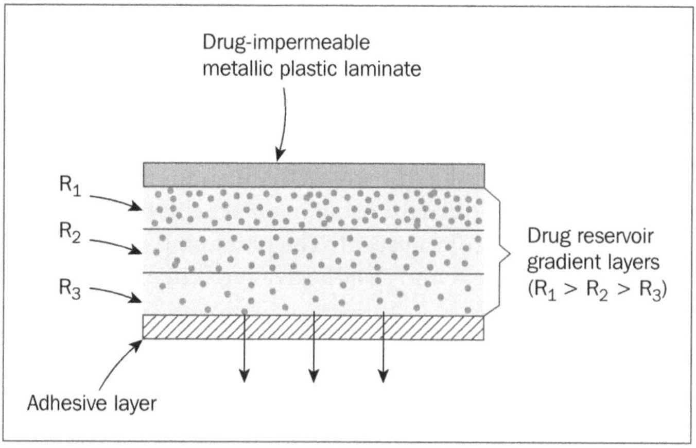

Catapres TTS and similar systems

We have discussed earlier that the physical robustness of a polymer matrix system reduces the risk of dose dumping, compared to a membrane permeation-controlled system, but does not usually lead to a zero-order release rate. In the example of Deponit we have seen one way to overcome this by using different layers of the matrix with different drug concentrations. In the Catapres transdermal controlled-release system polymer matrix diffusion had been combined with polymer membrane permeation control. The drug (clonidine) is dispersed in a polymer matrix but this is additionally covered by a polymer membrane that initially does not contain the drug. This polymer membrane controls the release of the drug and thus leads to zero-order release kinetics.

Other examples of polymer matrix systems combined with polymer membrane permeation control

- Transderm-Scop, which contains scopolamine as the active ingredient and also is a transdermal delivery system.
- Norplant II, which is a hybrid-type implant for the controlled release of levonorgestrel.

Nitrodisc system

This system is another variation on the simple polymer matrix system for transdermal controlled drug delivery. Here the drug is initially dispersed as a solid lactose trituration in a polyethylene glycol 400/water mixture. This dispersion is then finely dispersed in a polymer matrix (a silicone elastomer). Figure 6.9 shows a schematic of this system. Drug release follows a square root of time kinetics and 50 µg of nitroglycerine is released per cm^2 of the device per day.

Figure 6.9 Schematic of the Nitrodisc controlled drug delivery system.

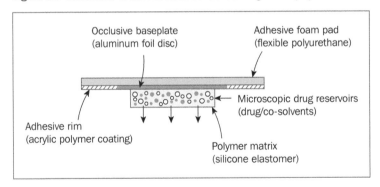

Activation-modulated controlled drug delivery systems

In previous sections we have discussed controlled drug delivery systems based on diffusion as the driving force for drug release. We have seen that this can be achieved by drug diffusion through a polymer membrane or through a

Tip

Other means of achieving controlled drug delivery have also been investigated but we will restrict ourselves here to methods that have led to successful marketed products. However other activation-modulated systems, for example based on vapour pressure activation, enzymatic or biochemical activation, sonophoresis and iontophoresis will continue to be investigated and will broaden the arsenal of methods available to achieve controlled drug delivery for a large number of drugs.

KeyPoints

- Osmosis is the diffusion of molecules from regions of high concentration to low concentration through a semipermeable membrane.
- If a drug delivery system has a semipermeable membrane that stops drugs diffusing out, water is drawn in.
- This water can then push the drug out of the delivery system through a delivery orifice.
- Drug release is then controlled by the semipermeable membrane properties and the osmotic pressure gradient.

polymer matrix. Diffusion, however, is not the only driving force that can be used to achieve controlled drug delivery. In this section we will discuss systems that use osmotic pressure, hydration and hydrolysis to achieve controlled drug delivery.

Osmotic pressure-activated controlled drug delivery systems

Osmosis is a process that is related to diffusion. Let us consider two solutions of different concentrations (for example, a high drug concentration of dissolved molecules or ions inside a drug delivery system, and a low concentration of dissolved molecules or ions outside the delivery system). If the inside and outside of the drug delivery system are separated by a semipermeable membrane, which is a membrane that is only permeable to solvent molecules but not to solute molecules, then the solvent will diffuse across the semipermeable membrane from the outside to the higher concentrated solution in the inside of the delivery system. This process is called osmosis and introduces an osmotic pressure in the inside of the delivery system. If such a system has a small release opening, the drug solution can be pushed out of the delivery system, leading to a controlled release of the drug.

It can be shown that the water influx (V/t) into such a system depends on:

- the surface area, thickness and water permeability of the semipermeable membrane (A_m, h_m and P_w respectively)
- the osmotic pressure difference inside and outside the drug delivery system ($\pi_i - \pi_o$):

$$\frac{V}{t} = \frac{A_m P_w}{h_m}(\pi_i - \pi_o)$$

From the above equation it can be seen that π needs to remain constant to achieve a zero-order release rate (all other factors in this equation can be regarded as constant). As the drug leaves the delivery system and water enters it, π_i, however, is only a constant if the solute concentration is maintained by dissolution of solids. This can be achieved by adding the drug as a solid dispersion to the delivery system. The resulting equation for drug release from such a system is:

$$\frac{Q}{t} = \frac{A_m P_w}{h_m}(\pi_i - \pi_o)C_s$$

where C_s is the saturation concentration of the drug in the inside of the delivery system.

Osmotic pressure-activated controlled drug delivery systems are mostly developed for oral drug delivery, and are also often called OROS (abbreviation for oral osmotic systems).

Elementary osmotic pumps

The simplest form of an oral osmotic system, the elementary osmotic pump, is shown in Figure 6.10. The drug is present in a tablet core that is coated with a semipermeable membrane. Into this membrane a small hole is drilled by a laser beam, and this acts as the delivery orifice. When such a system is ingested, water from the gastrointestinal tract will diffuse through the semipermeable membrane and will dissolve the drug, and the drug solution is pumped out through the drilled hole. The osmotic pressure controls the amount of dissolved drug that is pushed out into the gastrointestinal tract through the delivery orifice.

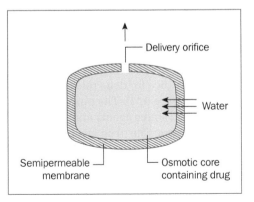

Delivery orifice

Water

Semipermeable membrane

Osmotic core containing drug

Figure 6.10 Schematic of an elementary osmotic pump.

For such a system to be useful, the drug has to be sufficiently water-soluble. To increase the osmotic pressure difference between the inside and outside of the delivery system $(\pi_i - \pi_o)$, other water-soluble excipients can be added.

Tip

Osmotic pressure is a colligative property. A colligative property is a property of a solution that depends only on the number of solute and solvent molecules (in other words, their molar ratio) but not the nature of the solute molecules. Colligative properties include vapour pressure lowering, boiling point elevation, freezing point depression and indeed osmotic pressure. It is therefore possible to increase the osmotic pressure difference by adding water-soluble, low-molecular-weight excipients such as sodium chloride or glucose to the inside of the osmotic drug delivery system.

This may be necessary if:

- the pharmacological activity of the drug is high and thus its required release rate is low
- solubility of the drug is insufficient to create a large enough osmotic pressure difference.

Example of an elementary osmotic pump

The Acutrim system is an example of a single-chamber oral osmotic controlled drug delivery system. The system consists of a tablet formulation of the drug phenyl propanolamine hydrochloride (PPA HCl). This drug is freely water-soluble and thus suitable for this type of controlled drug delivery. The tablet is coated with a semipermeable membrane (cellulose triacetate) with a laser beam-drilled orifice for release of the drug solution. To achieve an initially high drug release, the tablet is coated further with a thin layer of the drug that is dissolved immediately upon ingestion of the dosage form, before a constant release by the osmotic drug delivery system takes place. PPA HCl is used for appetite suppression and is released over a period of 16 h. This length of delivery is appropriate for an oral dosage form, given the transit time of the system in the gastrointestinal tract.

KeyPoints

- Push–pull systems comprise one push layer and one or more drug layers.
- In the gastrointestinal tract, water is drawn in, causing the push layer to swell and the formation of a liquid suspension in the drug layers.
- The expanding push layer pushes the drug suspension out of the exit hole drilled into the drug layer.

Push–pull systems

These systems are a further development of the elementary osmotic pump and are based on bilayer or trilayer tablets consisting of a push layer (which is drug-free) and other layer(s) containing the drug.

These multilayered tablets are again coated with a semipermeable membrane into which a small orifice for drug release has been drilled (Figure 6.11). The push layer contains osmotic active agents and water-swellable polymers. The drug layer contains the drug, osmotically active excipients and suspending agents.

Upon ingestion, water from the gastrointestinal tract will enter the system, leading to:

- swelling of the push layer
- formation of a liquid suspension of the drug in the drug layer(s).

The expanding push layer will then lead to the release of the drug in suspended form into the gastrointestinal tract. It is thus necessary that the drug dissolves after release from the push–pull system.

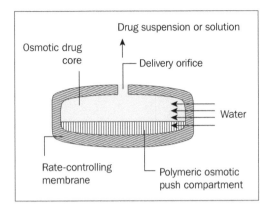

Figure 6.11 Schematic of a push–pull system.

Osmotic drug core

Drug suspension or solution

Delivery orifice

Water

Rate-controlling membrane

Polymeric osmotic push compartment

Examples of oral push–pull systems

- Procardia XL: the drug (indometacin) is present in a drug layer and is released as a drug suspension at a constant rate for 24 h independent of pH or gastrointestinal motility.
- Ditropan XL: this system contains oxybutynin chloride in the drug layer. Oxybutyrin is an antispasmodic, anticholinergic agent for the control of overactive bladder.
- Dynacirc CR: this system contains the calcium channel blocker isradipine used to treat high blood pressure.
- Glucotrol XL: this system contains glipizide, an oral blood-glucose-lowering agent.
- Covera HS: this system has been designed to initiate the release of the active verapamil hydrochloride 4–5 h after ingestion. This has been achieved by the introduction of a drug-free layer between the core and outer semipermeable membrane. Water from the gastrointestinal tract enters the tablet and the delay layer is solubilised. As tablet hydration continues, the push layer expands and pushes against the drug layer, releasing the drug. Covera HS is taken in the evening, leading to peak drug concentration in the early hours of the day. The medication is used in the management of cardiovascular diseases. Likelihood of a stroke is highest in the early hours of the day.
- Concerta is an OROS system in which the drug methylphenidate (for the treatment of attention deficit hyperactivity disorder) is present in two layers. To achieve an initial high dose of the drug, the tablet is also coated with a thin layer of the drug that is dissolved immediately upon ingestion of the dosage form. This leads to approximately 20% of the dose being released in the first hour. Methylphenidate is then released from the two drug layers for approximately 12 h.

Push–pull systems can also be used for administration by other than the oral route. The Alzet osmotic pump is an example of an insertable or implantable device with osmotically controlled release of the drug. Figure 6.12 shows a schematic of this device. The drug

Figure 6.12 Schematic of an
Alzet osmotic pump.

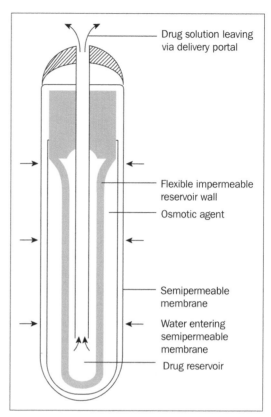

Drug solution leaving
via delivery portal

Flexible impermeable
reservoir wall

Osmotic agent

Semipermeable
membrane

Water entering
semipermeable
membrane

Drug reservoir

is usually present in solution in a reservoir bag with a flexible, impermeable wall. This reservoir is surrounded by another reservoir, containing the osmotically active agents which are again surrounded by a semipermeable membrane. Upon insertion, for example in the rectal cavity, or implantation into the body, water from the surrounding tissues will penetrate through the semipermeable wall and dissolve the osmotically active agents, thus increasing the osmotic pressure. This will create a pressure on the collapsible drug reservoir, reducing its volume and forcing the drug out of the reservoir through a delivery opening. Controlled zero-order release can be obtained for days or weeks.

KeyPoint

- Hydrophilic polymer matrices which swell on contact with water offer hydration-activated controlled release.

Hydration-activated controlled drug delivery systems

These systems contain hydrophilic polymers into which a drug is dispersed. Once the system comes into contact with fluid, for example in the stomach after oral administration or from surrounding tissues after implantation, the polymer matrix swells and this swelling allows for release of the drug. An example of these systems is Valrelease tablets, which were discussed in Chapter 5.

Hydrolysis-activated controlled drug delivery systems

Whilst the above-mentioned hydrocolloids are swellable systems, other polymers are bioerodible or biodegradable. Polylactides, poly(lactide co-glycolide) copolymers and poly(orthoesters) belong in this group of polymers. We discussed these polymers in Chapter 5.

However, the following three examples belong in the group of controlled-release systems.

Biodegradable controlled-release systems

Biodegradable polymers can be exploited for controlled release in a range of formulations.

- *Implants*. Zoladex is a cylindrical subcutaneous poly(lactide co-glycolide) copolymer implant containing the drug goserelin. The drug (a gonadtrophin-releasing hormone analogue used in the treatment of prostate cancer) is released from the implant over a period of up to 3 months initially through surface erosion of the polymer and in a second phase though bulk erosion. The hydrolytic degradation of the polymer chains controls the release of the drug.
- *Controlled-release microspheres*. Lupron Depot is an injectable formulation. The drug (luprolide, again a gonadotrophin-releasing hormone analogue used in the treatment of prostate cancer and endometriosis) is incorporated into microspheres (polylactic acid), which are injected subcutaneously. The drug is released in a controlled fashion for up to 4 months.
- *Controlled-release wafers*. Gliadel is a controlled-release wafer for local drug release in a surgical cavity after resection of a brain tumour. The active ingredient in the wafer is the oncolytic drug carmustine. The drug is incorporated in a biodegradable polyanhydride copolymer called polifeprosan 20, which chemically is a random block copolymer of *bis*(*p*-carboxyphenoxy) propane and sebacic acid at a molar ratio of 2:8. The chemical structure of this copolymer is shown in Figure 6.13. The drug is released by biodegradation and bioerosion of the copolymer after the wafer comes into contact with the aqueous environment of the surgical cavity, by hydrolysis of the anhydride bonds. It has been found that approximately 70% of

Figure 6.13 Chemical structure of polifeprosan 20.

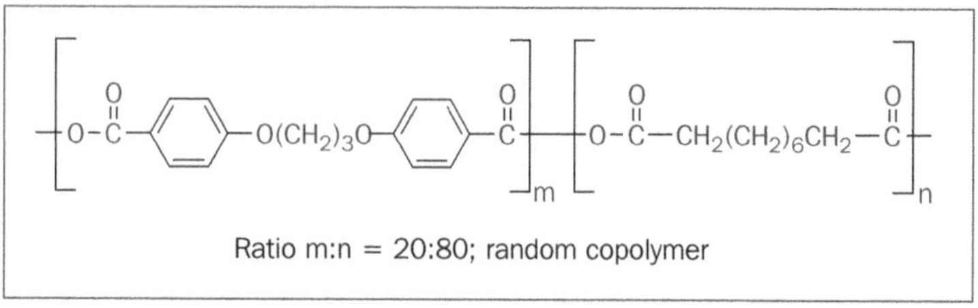

$$\left[O - \overset{\overset{O}{\|}}{C} - \bigcirc - O(CH_2)_3O - \bigcirc - \overset{\overset{O}{\|}}{C} \right]_m \left[O - \overset{\overset{O}{\|}}{C} - CH_2(CH_2)_6CH_2 - \overset{\overset{O}{\|}}{C} \right]_n$$

Ratio m:n = 20:80; random copolymer

the copolymer degrades within a period of 3 weeks, leading to a controlled release of the drug. The degradation products of the polymer are renally excreted (carboxyphenoxy propane) or metabolised in the liver (sebacic acid is a dicarboxylic fatty acid, naturally occurring in the body). Up to eight of these wafers are inserted into the surgical cavity after the operation.

Polymers based on PLGA-PEG-PLGA units (triblock copolymers) are biodegradable and also show unique thermo-reversible properties: at ambient temperature the polymer is water-soluble but forms a water-insoluble gel at body temperature (i.e. above the critical gelation temperature). The sol–gel transition is due to the rearrangement of the hydrophobic and hydrophilic polymer chains in response to a change in temperature (Figure 6.14). This results in a gel that is several orders of magnitude more viscous than the sol and serves as a drug depot enabling controlled drug release for 1–6 weeks upon degradation of the gel. Furthermore, poorly water-soluble drugs may be solubilised in the hydrophobic cavities of the polymer. Additional benefits of the polymer are the potential protection and stabilisation of sensitive compounds such as proteins. When injected into the tumour tissue the efficacy of a triblock copolymer/paclitaxel combination (OncoGel) offered comparable efficacy at doses 10-fold lower than the maximum tolerated systemic dosing of paclitaxel.

Fully esterified sucrose derivatives (sucrose acetate isobutyrate, SAIB) have also been considered for the formulation of controlled drug release. After mixing SAIB with the drug and one or more additives (such as pharmaceutically acceptable solvents), the viscous

Figure 6.14 Sol–gel transition due to the rearrangement of the hydrophobic and hydrophilic polymer chains of PLGA-PEG-PLGA triblock copolymers in response to a change in temperature.

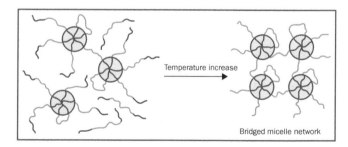

Temperature increase

Bridged micelle network

liquid SAIB is injected subcutaneously, generating a highly viscous depot (SABER) from which the drug is slowly delivered for time periods ranging from 1 day to 3 months. Drug release can be tailored by the appropriate choice and amount of additives. Injectable SABER formulations are currently investigated in clinical trials for the delivery of the antipsychotic risperidone (Relday) and the local anaesthetic bupivacaine (Posidur). It should be noted that the same technology can also be employed for the development of sustained-release oral products.

Feedback-regulated controlled drug delivery systems

A constant plasma concentration of the drug is not always desirable and instead a pulsatile release may be required, for example for the treatment of hormonally controlled disorders. Another key example is insulin delivery to diabetic patients; this would strongly benefit

> **KeyPoints**
>
> - A constant plasma profile is not always wanted.
> - Delivery systems which could release drugs in response to biological feedback are currently being investigated.

from a long-term but variable release of the drug according to the blood glucose level. Research is under way to develop bioresponsive delivery systems for such situations. In these systems a biological feedback is used to regulate the drug release. In the case of feedback-regulated insulin release this is the glucose concentration. Currently such systems are not available on the market.

Insulin has been encapsulated in a polymeric hydrogel shell containing tertiary amino groups. The shell additionally contains glucose oxidase. At high pH the polymer is insoluble and does not swell, thus it does not allow for insulin to be released. If, however, the glucose concentration is rising, glucose is increasingly penetrating into the polymer. Here the oxidase will oxidise the glucose molecules to gluconic acid, thus lowering the pH in the membrane. This leads to a protonation of the tertiary amino groups to quaternary ammonium groups, which in turn will render the polymer more hydrophilic, allowing it to swell and leading to the release of the encapsulated insulin. This is shown schematically in Figure 6.15.

Another way of feedback-regulated insulin delivery is the MiniMed Paradigm Veo insulin pump, an insulin pump together with continuous glucose monitoring. Here, a glucose sensor, which is placed in the hypodermic tissue, continuously measures the glucose level and electronically sends this data to an insulin pump. In this manner, the pump can then deliver the required insulin dose at every given time point. To prevent hypoglycaemic situations the sensor also stops the insulin feed in case of low sugar levels.

Figure 6.15 Schematic of a feedback-regulated insulin delivery system. See text for details.

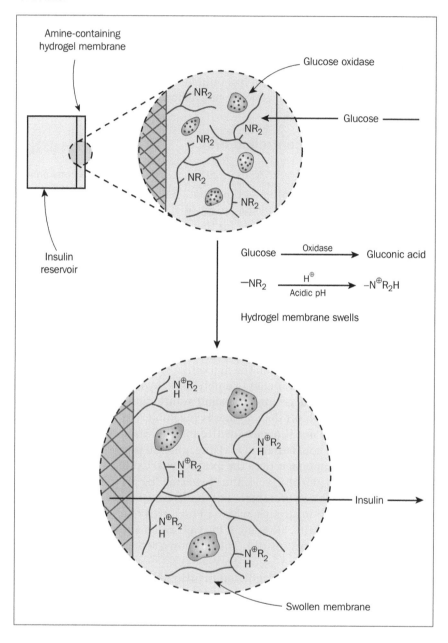

Conclusions

Steady-state plasma concentrations can be achieved by drug infusions. However these are not convenient. Controlled-release drug delivery systems can be formulated to give reproducible release kinetics and predicable drug plasma concentrations similar to infusions. Controlled release can be achieved by controlling diffusion, osmosis, hydration or hydrolysis. These systems can offer controlled release but do not target and retain the drug at the site of action. Methods to promote drug targeting will be discussed in Chapter 7.

Self-assessment

After having read this chapter you should be able to:
- compare and contrast sustained- and controlled-release dosage forms
- draw an idealised plasma concentration versus time profile of a drug after IV injection and infusion
- list the advantages of controlled-release dosage forms over conventional delivery systems
- draw an idealised plasma concentration versus time profile of a drug delivered in several doses of an oral immediate-release dosage form and a controlled-release dosage form
- explain what is meant by a polymer membrane permeation-controlled system and discuss its advantages and disadvantages
- give examples of polymer membrane permeation-controlled drug delivery systems on the market
- compare and contrast polymer matrix diffusion-controlled systems with polymer membrane permeation-controlled systems, list their advantages and disadvantages and draw their typical drug release profiles
- give examples of polymer matrix diffusion-controlled drug delivery systems on the market
- explain the physicochemical basis of osmotic pressure-activated controlled drug delivery systems
- explain the principle and draw a schematic of a push–pull system
- give examples of OROS on the market
- explain the principle of hydrolysis-activated controlled drug delivery systems
- give examples of hydrolysis-activated controlled drug delivery systems on the market.

Questions

1. **Indicate which of the following statements is/are correct (there may be more than one answer).**
    Whilst drug infusions can provide controlled plasma levels, they have a range of disadvantages, including:
    a. Inconvenience for the patient.
    b. Necessity for medical personnel to be involved in the administration.
    c. Requirement for frequently repeated administration.
    d. Cannot be used for infants and elderly.
    e. Requirement for a sterile formulation.

2. **Indicate which of the following statements is/are correct (there may be more than one answer).**
    a. Using a controlled-release dosage form, drug plasma concentrations are predictable but the desired drug level may only be maintained for a short period of time.
    b. Using a controlled-release dosage form may decrease times of subtherapeutic drug concentrations and thus ineffective treatment.
    c. Using a controlled-release dosage form may decrease times of a too high drug concentration that may lead to avoidable side-effects.
    d. Drugs that benefit from delivery by controlled-release systems include those used for treatment of diseases where variable plasma concentrations are required, such as diabetes.
    e. Controlled-release dosage forms have only been developed for oral administration.

3. **Indicate which of the following statements is/are correct (there may be more than one answer).**
    a. Drug release from polymer membrane permeation systems is controlled by chemical degradation of the polymer.
    b. Polymer membrane permeation systems comprise a drug reservoir within a polymeric coating.
    c. The polymer coating of a polymer membrane permeation system has to be non-porous.
    d. Drug release from polymer membrane permeation systems is dependent on the drug concentration in the reservoir, the physicochemical properties of the drug and the properties of the polymer membrane.
    e. Whilst conventional dosage forms are characterised by a dose (for example, 100 mg of drug per tablet), controlled-release delivery systems are characterised by a release rate (for example, 20 µg of drug released per hour).

4. **Indicate which of the following statements is/are correct (there may be more than one answer).**
a. Ocusert is a controlled-release drug delivery system fabricated as an ocular insert.
b. In the Ocusert system the drug (pilocarpine) is present in the reservoir as a drug–alginate complex.
c. To facilitate localisation of the Ocusert system in the eye, the delivery system contains a white titanium dioxide ring.
d. The polymer membrane of Ocusert is a non-porous ethylene vinyl acetate copolymer.
e. Several Ocusert systems have been designed with release rates of 20 or 40 mg pilocarpine/h. The systems can be used for 4 or 7 weeks for the treatment of glaucoma.

5. **Indicate which of the following statements is/are correct (there may be more than one answer).**
a. For controlled transdermal drug delivery the drugs should ideally penetrate easily though the stratum corneum of the skin.
b. For controlled transdermal drug delivery the drugs should have a high molecular weight.
c. For controlled transdermal drug delivery the drugs should be fairly hydrophilic.
d. As the stratum corneum of the skin is a very good barrier for absorption, this limits the number of suitable drugs for controlled release via this route.

6. **Indicate which of the following statements is/are correct (there may be more than one answer).**
a. For polymer matrix drug delivery systems, release is controlled by drug diffusion through the polymer matrix.
b. For polymer matrix systems drug delivery systems always require an additional polymer coating.
c. Polymer matrix drug delivery systems can be subdivided, e.g. patches can be cut.
d. Polymer matrix drug delivery systems generally give rise to linear release profiles of the drug as a function of the cube root of time.

7. **Indicate which of the following statements is/are correct (there may be more than one answer).**
a. The Nitrodisc system is an example of a polymer matrix system for transdermal controlled drug delivery.
b. In the Nitrodisc system the drug is initially dispersed as a solid lactose trituration in a polyethylene glycol 400/water mixture.
c. The dispersion described in **b** is then finely dispersed in a polymer matrix (a silicone elastomer).

d. Drug release follows a square root of time kinetics and 50 mg of nitroglycerine is released per cm² of the device per day.

8. **Indicate which of the following statements is/are correct (there may be more than one answer).**
    The equation for drug release from osmotic pressure-activated controlled drug delivery systems is:

$$\frac{Q}{t} = \frac{A_m P_w}{h_m}(\pi_i - \pi_o)C_s$$

In this equation:
a. Q/t is the amount of drug released per time.
b. A_m is the surface area of the semipermeable membrane.
c. P_w is the drug permeability of the semipermeable membrane.
d. h_m is the thickness of the semipermeable membrane.
e. $(\pi_i - \pi_o)$ is the osmotic pressure difference inside and outside the drug delivery system.
f. C_s is the saturation concentration of the drug in the outside of the delivery system.

9. **Indicate which of the following statements is/are correct (there may be more than one answer).**
a. Zoladex is an example of a biodegradable controlled drug delivery system.
b. Zoladex is a cylindrical subcutaneous poly(lactide co-glycolide) copolymer implant containing the drug goserelin.
c. In Zoladex the drug is released from the implant over a period of up to 3 days.
d. In Zoladex the hydrolytic degradation of the polymer chains controls the release of the drug.
e. In Zoladex drug release is achieved initially through bulk erosion of the polymer and in a second phase through surface erosion.

Reference

Attwood D, Florence AT (2008) *Fasttrack Physical Pharmacy.* London: Pharmaceutical Press.

Further reading

General
Baker RW (1987) *Controlled Release of Biologically Active Agents.* New York: Wiley-Interscience.
Chien YW (1991) *Novel Drug Delivery Systems.* London: Informa Healthcare.

Kydonieus AF (1991) *Treatise on Controlled Drug Delivery: Fundamentals, Optimization, Applications.* London: Informa Healthcare.

Li X (2005) *Design of Controlled Release Drug Delivery Systems.* New York, NY: McGraw Hill.

Robinson JR, Lee VHL (1987) *Controlled Drug Delivery: Fundamentals and Applications.* London: Informa Healthcare.

Remington's Science and Practice of Pharmacy (2006) 21st edn. Philadelphia, PA: Lippincott Williams and Wilkins.

Sinko PJ (2006) *Martin's Physical Pharmacy and Pharmaceutical Sciences,* 5th edn. Philadelphia, PA: Lippincott Williams and Wilkins.

Oral osmotic systems

Wong PSL *et al.* (2002) Osmotically controlled tablets. In: Rathbone M (ed.) *Modified-Release Drug Delivery Technology.* New York, NY: Marcel Dekker, pp. 101–105.

chapter 7
Site-directed drug targeting

Overview

In this chapter we will:

- define drug targeting
- identify potential targets for drug delivery
- describe the barriers to drug delivery
- discuss the different attributes of passive and active targeting
- discuss how targeting systems may enter cells to reach intracellular targets.

General principles of drug targeting

In the previous chapters we have discussed how we can control the release of drugs from delivery systems. However after entering the systemic circulation most drugs distribute freely throughout the body. Rate-controlling systems can dictate the rate of drug delivery but in general they do not control the fate of the drug once the drug enters the body. Drug targeting aims to control the distribution of a drug within the body such that the majority of the dose selectively interacts with the target tissue at a cellular or subcellular level. Simply, we want to direct the drug specifically to where its activity is required, at the optimum concentration, for the desired time. By doing so, we can enhance the activity and specificity of the drug and reduce its toxicity, thereby improving its therapeutic profile.

For example, drug targeting can improve the outcome of chemotherapy by:

- promoting the distribution of a chemotherapeutic drug to cancer cells, thus enhancing potency

KeyPoints

- The biodistribution of a drug may be controlled using a drug-targeting system that can control the localisation and release of a drug, thereby enhancing its potency and reducing toxicity.
- This can also help to protect the drug from inactivation before it reaches its target.

Tip

There are a range of chemotherapeutic drugs available, which have various mechanisms of action. However all chemotherapy works by destroying cells and chemotherapeutic drugs therefore are inherently highly toxic with a narrow therapeutic window. Targeting of these drugs can greatly improve the side-effect profile of these medicines.

- enhancing the amount of drug that acts solely in cancer cells, thus reducing toxicity to non-cancerous cells
- prolonging the retention of the chemotherapeutic drug at the tumour site.

Requirements for effective drug targeting

We have already seen in the previous chapters that the route by which a drug formulation is administered can have a strong impact on the rate of drug delivery and its site of action. Indeed, targeting of specific organs can be achieved if the organ is accessible from the external environment, for example by the delivery of drops to the eye, inhalation of dry powders to the lung, application of creams to the skin. However, directing a drug to a site of action via the route of administration does not ensure drug retention at this site; systemic drug absorption can occur after delivery via a variety of routes. The situation becomes even more complicated if we want to reach internal organs exclusively, such as the brain, liver and kidneys, or tissue sites, such as certain tumours. To reach these sites the drug must leave the systemic circulation and specifically accumulate at targets inside the body. Local delivery to internal organs and tissues can be achieved by physical means such as direct injection (e.g. intratumour injection) or using implants (e.g. Gliadel, a polymer wafer that releases the drug when placed in the brain: see Chapter 6). However, again this does not ensure precise targeting and retention at the required site. In addition, most drugs do not possess the required physicochemical characteristics to enter target cells, so mechanisms to achieve this must be considered in the design of a targeting system if intracellular delivery is required.

Therefore, there are a range of requirements that an effective drug-targeting system must ideally offer:

- There must be no non-specific interactions with biological components/tissues/organs.
- The targeting system should be non-toxic/therapeutically acceptable.
- It should specifically target the drug to the physiological target.
- It should retain the drug during transit the site.
- The drug must be able to access the target site.
- The drug should be retained at the site.
- The drug must be released from its delivery system.

Tip

Dr Paul Ehrlich (1854–1915), a German scientist, developed the concept of the 'magic bullet' which was based on the idea that compounds could be designed to target disease causing organisms selectively, thereby killing only the targeted organism. His ideas were based on the selective staining of bacteria and certain tissues in histology.

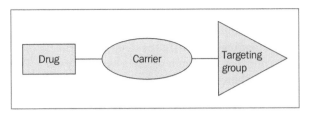

Figure 7.1 Schematic representation of a drug carrier-targeting device.

To achieve site-specific delivery of a drug, an effective targeting system may comprise drug, carrier and targeting group (Figure 7.1).

Consideration of the drug being delivered

Not all drug therapies can be improved with drug targeting. For example, drugs that have the same site of efficacy and toxicity will not gain from this approach. With regard to their pharmacokinetics, drugs with high total clearance are generally more appropriate for targeting since drug not retained at the target site will be cleared rapidly.

Consideration of the drug target

The choice of targeting strategy for a drug is clearly dependent on what the target is, and what its key attributes are. There are various sites and levels to which we can target a drug, including:

- Specific organs: examples include targeting the brain to treat Alzheimer's, Parkinson's and Creutzfeldt–Jakob disease or targeting the lung in the treatment of cystic fibrosis.
- Tissues: examples include targeting tumours or sites of inflammation.
- Invading organisms: for example, targeting bacteria, viruses and parasites (tuberculosis, human immunodeficiency virus (HIV) and malaria).
- Specific cells: for example, targeting of trastuzumab to human epidermal growth factor receptor-2 (HER2) + cancer cells.
- Cytosolic targets: many drugs require delivery across the cell membrane since their specific target is inside the cell. For example, within the cytoplasm, proteins or receptors (e.g. glucocorticoid receptors) may be the target.
- Subcellular compartments: additional compartments within the cell, such as the nucleus, or organelles, such as mitochondria, may also contain the target, e.g. targeting of DNA for intercalating agents such as doxorubicin, or for gene therapy applications.

As we progress through these levels of targeting, the level of specificity that we can achieve is improved; however the barriers that must be overcome are also enhanced.

> ## KeyPoints
>
> - Most drugs interact with a cellular constituent to exert their action. However what is the designated target will depend on the pharmacological action required.
> - The target site may be a specific organ, a distinct population of cells or an intracellular target.

Key Points

- The physicochemical nature of a drug carrier system can dictate the fate and distribution of the drug.
- Movement out of the systemic circulation is required for drugs to reach many target sites.

The drug delivery system

To reach a desired target we can either chemically modify the drug using the prodrug approach or use a carrier system. The attributes of the various carrier systems will be discussed in detail in Chapter 8. There are two general classes of carrier systems:

1. Soluble carrier systems:
   a. Includes natural and synthetic water-soluble polymers and antibodies.
   b. With these systems the drug is conjugated to the carrier.
2. Particulate carrier systems:
   a. Includes liposomes, microspheres and nanoparticles.
   b. Here the drug is either surface-bound or entrapped within the carrier.

In principle, there is little difference between prodrugs and drug–carrier conjugates: both have the active drug administered as part of a larger molecule that has pharmacokinetic and pharmacodynamic properties that are generally different from that of the active drug. However, the pharmacokinetic properties of a prodrug and a drug–carrier conjugate will be quite different due to their different physicochemical properties (e.g. molecular weight, molecular shape, hydrophilic/hydrophobic properties), with drug–carrier conjugates being larger and, as such, they can be considered as macromolecular/colloidal drug delivery systems.

Depending on the physiology of the target, these systems may naturally accumulate at the target site (this is known as passive targeting). Alternatively the system may be actively targeted to a site using a target-specific recognition component. For example, the addition of galactose groups to a carrier system can promote targeting of galactose receptors on the surface of liver parenchymal cells. However it is important to recognise that such a targeted system is not a 'homing device' which would purposely search out the target; rather these systems still rely on random encounters of the delivery system with its appropriate target during its transit through the body.

As discussed, to reach internal organs the drug must leave the central circulation by crossing the endothelium. Current drug-targeting systems based on the outline above are generally developed for administration via the parenteral route. However drug delivery systems entering the systemic circulation are confronted with an assortment of chemical, physical and immunological barriers in the body. These are designed to

Tip

The endothelium controls the movement of white blood cells and other material in and out of the blood. The nature of this lining varies with the organ type, with some being more permeable in nature (e.g. in the kidneys) than others (e.g. in the brain) depending on the organ function. To access such organs, the delivery system must be able to cross this barrier.

prevent foreign substances, such as drugs and delivery systems, from entering further into the body via the systemic circulation.

Physiological and biological barriers to drug targeting

Often drugs are designed to have a relatively low molecular weight and to have a balance between hydrophobicity and hydrophilicity to allow them to partition across lipid membranes relatively easily, yet still have sufficient water solubility. Therefore, without the aid of the delivery system, a drug within the systemic circulation can be rapidly distributed throughout the body, reaching non-target sites, and it will be quickly metabolised by the liver and/or rapidly excreted via the kidneys. By contrast, drug carrier systems are much larger than the active drug and they are not able to partition across the endothelium. Therefore they tend to have different biodistribution profiles than the parent drug and are retained within different compartments within the body. For effective targeting, it is essential that a drug-targeting system is not cleared too quickly, and ideally the targeting delivery system will provide a pharmacokinetic profile which will allow the drug to interact with its physiological target, such as a receptor. Indeed, we should bear in mind that the circulation half-life of the system must be appropriate to allow random encounters of the delivery system with such targets. Therefore we need to camouflage the drug and its carrier from the systemic environment until the drug reaches its target.

> **KeyPoints**
>
> - The body's natural defence system has a range of methods to remove particulate drug delivery systems and drug conjugates.
> - Molecules within the blood can bind to particulates and mark them for recognition and destruction by phagocytic cells within the immune system.

A summary of the elimination processes faced by a delivery system in systemic circulation is shown in Figure 7.2. From this figure we see that we must offset the rate of delivery of the drug to the target site against the removal of the drug carrier from the body and removal of the free drug from the target site. Further we should bear in mind that the actual physiological target may be intracellular and therefore additional rates of transport across cell membranes may need to be accounted for.

Elimination of the drug carrier

If the drug carrier system is removed too quickly from the circulation an effective drug concentration at the target site may not be reached. Unlike free drugs, drug carrier systems are generally too large to be eliminated by the kidney as clearance through kidney excretion is limited to sizes below 10 nm. However the body has various mechanisms to support the removal of larger macromolecules and particulates from the body, including clearance by the mononuclear phagocyte system and opsonisation.

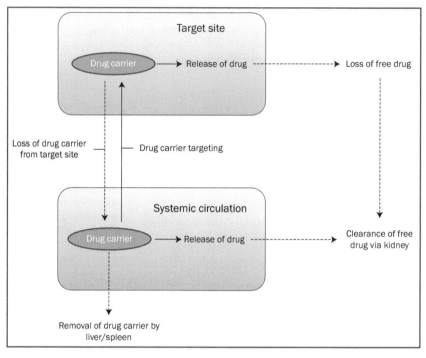

Figure 7.2 Routes of elimination of a drug and a drug delivery system.

KeyPoint

To avoid recognition and removal of particulate drug delivery systems from the systemic circulation the particles should be formulated to be less than 100 nm in size, and have a hydrophilic surface.

A major barrier that drug delivery systems must be able to overcome in the systemic circulation is the removal of particulates by phagocytic cells of the mononuclear phagocyte system (MPS). The MPS consists of cells, including bone marrow monoblasts, blood monocytes, mobile tissue macrophages and fixed tissue macrophages such as those found in the liver (Kupffer cells), the lung (alveolar macrophages), the spleen, bone marrow and lymph nodes. The main function of these phagocytic cells is to eliminate and remove foreign material, including bacteria and proteins. The phagocytic activity of these cells is mediated by immunoglobulin binding and binding by other marker molecules found in serum. They are also involved in antigen processing and presentation as part of the immune response. When injected intravenously, particles can be quickly cleared from the circulation by the liver and spleen macrophages. Therefore the MPS presents a significant barrier to effective drug targeting since it has the ability to filter out and destroy a drug delivery system unless appropriate formulation approaches are used to avoid this.

Tip

The MPS is sometimes also referred to as the reticuloendothelial system, although this is now generally seen as an obsolete term.

Recognition of the carriers: opsonisation

Whilst within the central compartment of the body (blood and lymph), a drug delivery system is in an aqueous polar medium, which contains a variety of molecules and macromolecules. This polar medium and the molecules dissolved therein can interact non-covalently with drugs and their carriers through electrostatic and hydrogen-bonding interactions.

Therefore the delivery system should be designed to avoid these interactions which can lead to the possible detection and clearance of the delivery system from the systemic circulation. In particular, opsonisation of the drug and/or its carrier must be avoided. This is a process where the surface of a particle or pathogen is coated by molecules (known as opsonins). The opsonisation of foreign particles, such as bacteria and particulate drug carriers, is a method of marking the particulates for easier recognition and destruction by phagocytes. The phagocytosis of these 'tagged particles' is enhanced because phagocytes carry surface receptors that bind to the opsonins and the foreign particle is engulfed, surrounded, phagocytosed and ultimately digested in the various lysosomal compartments within the cells.

There are a range of blood opsonic factors, including fibronectin, antibodies and complement proteins. In terms of particulate drug delivery systems, the complement component 3b is the most significant as it non-specifically attaches to particulate surfaces and triggers the recognition and ultimate destruction of these systems. Antibodies (in particular, immunoglobulin (Ig) G) also act as opsonins by binding to sites through their Fab region, leaving the Fc region free. Phagocytes have Fc receptors and therefore bind to the coated molecule or particulate and internalise and destroy it.

Tips

Antibodies, also known as immunoglobulins, are produced by B cells and can bind to bacteria and viruses. They have a structure similar in nature to the letter 'Y'. The tip of the Y is the Fab region and binds antigens (fragment, antigen binding). The base of the 'Y' is the Fc (fragment, crystallisable) region.

There are also around 20 different complement proteins: these are generally small in size and mainly produced by the liver.

Important factors in opsonisation and clearance

Suppression of opsonisation and avoiding MPS recognition and receptor-mediated phagocytosis are primary concerns when designing a drug-targeting system. Key factors which play an important role in opsonisation and MPS recognition are:

- Particle size: most particles are subject to clearance by macrophages of the MPS regardless of their size. To avoid MPS uptake, sizes below 100 nm are preferred but their surface characteristics must also be considered. Maximal phagocytosis by the MPS occurs with particles around 1–2 µm, whilst large particulates over 5–6 µm tend to become trapped in the lung capillaries.

Tip

PEG is also known as poly(ethylene oxide) or polyoxyethylene and has the general structure of $HO-CH_2-(CH_2-O-CH_2-)_n-CH_2-OH$.

Tips

Cells, organs and molecules of the immune system

Monocytes: white blood cells with a bean-shaped nucleus. They are the precursors of tissue macrophages.

Macrophages: large mononuclear phagocytic cells found in most tissues involved in stimulating the immune system. These are the mature forms of monocytes that have left the blood and entered the tissue.

Phagocytic cells: cells able to internalise particulate matter, such as bacteria, by endocytosis. The main groups of phagocytic cells are neutrophils and macrophages.

Kupffer cells: macrophage cells prevalent in the liver.

Lymphoid organs: organised tissue that contains a large number of lymphocytes. The thymus and bone marrow are primary lymphoid organs where lymphocytes are generated. The main secondary lymphoid tissues are the lymph nodes, spleen and mucosa-associated lymphoid tissues such as tonsils, Peyer's patches and the appendix. This is where immune responses are initiated.

Opsonins: molecules that bind to pathogens and particles and facilitate their phagocytosis. These include fibronectin, immunoglobulins and complement proteins.

Opsonisation: the coating of a pathogen or other particle with a molecule that makes it more readily recognised and phagocytosed.

- Surface charge: neutral systems tend to remain longer in circulation compared to their charged counterparts. In particular cationic systems quickly interact with various components whilst in systemic circulation and are rapidly filtered out by the MPS.
- Surface hydrophilicity: adding a hydrophilic polymer coat to a carrier system reduces protein adsorption and opsonisation, thus suppressing macrophage recognition. Poly(ethyleneglycol) (PEG) coating is commonly used to achieve this effect and is employed clinically in the liposomal drug delivery system Caelyx/doxil (Chapter 8). This PEG coating is sometimes referred to as steric stabilisation, 'stealth' coating or PEGylation. The ability of PEG to protect against opsonisation is thought to result from the local concentration of highly hydrated groups of PEG which sterically inhibit hydrophobic and electrostatic interactions with the various blood opsonins. PEG is particularly useful in this regard as it has good solubility in aqueous media, the polymer chains are very flexible and it has very low toxicity, antigenicity and immunogenicity. Furthermore it is non-biodegradable, does not form any metabolites and does not accumulate in MPS cells. PEG is used in several clinical products; however several other polymers have been shown to offer the same sterically stabilising effect. The efficiency of the hydrophilic polymer coat to mask the system from recognition is a function of the polymer used, and the polymer's length, shape and surface density on the carrier.

Therefore to avoid MPS uptake and rapid clearance from the circulation delivery systems should be formulated:

- to be below 100 nm in size
- to have a modified surface to minimise opsonisation, e.g. PEG-coated.

Escape from the systemic circulation

Whilst clearance of a drug delivery system is a major concern, drug delivery systems that circumvent recognition by the MPS do not necessarily offer the solution to drug targeting. Prolonged circulation is ideal for slow or controlled release of therapeutic agents or in the treatment of vascular disorders and in vascular imaging. However, a long circulation profile does not ensure effective targeting. The delivery system generally needs to leave the vasculature before it can reach its target. This requires the system to cross the endothelial lining of the blood circulation. The structure of the blood capillary wall is complex and varies in different organs and tissues. We can differentiate between three types of capillaries with respect to their endothelial lining (Figure 7.3):

1. Continuous: these are common and widely distributed in the body. They have tight junctions between the endothelial cells and a continuous basement membrane (e.g. capillaries in the brain, lung and muscles).
2. Fenestrated: these have gaps of between 20 and 80 nm between the endothelial cells (e.g. capillaries in the kidney, and gastrointestinal tract).
3. Sinusoidal: here the endothelial cells have gaps of up to 150 nm between them and the basement membrane is either discontinuous (e.g. in the spleen) or absent (e.g. in the liver).

In most parts of the body the endothelial lining is continuous and the endothelial cells are situated on a basal membrane with tight junctions between adjacent cells. Macromolecules can cross this endothelium by passive processes; however transport across the

Figure 7.3 Representation of the various types of capillaries with respect to their endothelial lining.

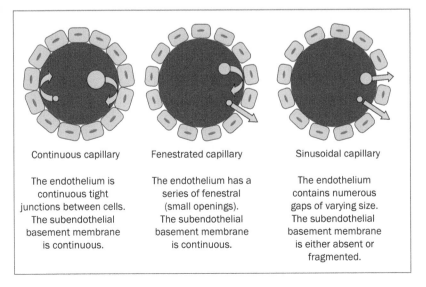

Continuous capillary	Fenestrated capillary	Sinusoidal capillary
The endothelium is continuous tight junctions between cells. The subendothelial basement membrane is continuous.	The endothelium has a series of fenestral (small openings). The subendothelial basement membrane is continuous.	The endothelium contains numerous gaps of varying size. The subendothelial basement membrane is either absent or fragmented.

endothelium decreases with increasing molecular size. Therefore, for drug delivery systems their escape from the circulation is normally restricted to sites where the endothelial lining is fenestrated or sinusoidal and has a number of gaps between the cells. This resembles the structure of capillaries within the liver, spleen and bone marrow, or where the integrity of the endothelial barrier has been disturbed by inflammatory processes or by tumour growth. In the liver, the size of the gaps can be as large as 150 nm. At sites of inflammation the endothelial fenestrations can be as large as 200 nm and in tumour capillaries they are generally no larger than 300 nm.

KeyPoints

- There are two main types of targeting: passive targeting and active targeting.
- Passive targeting exploits the natural conditions of the target organ to direct the drug to the target site.
- Active targeting uses targeting groups such as antibodies to bind to specific receptors on cells.

Types of drug targeting

The mechanism by which a drug delivery system is targeted can be divided into two main types:

1. Passive targeting. The distribution of the carrier is dictated by the local physiological conditions or by the MPS.
2. Active targeting. The distribution of the carrier is dictated by interactions between a ligand and its associated receptor.

Passive targeting

Passive targeting is the mechanism by which we take advantage of the natural pathological conditions of our target to allow the preferential accumulation of drug carrier at the target site.

Passive targeting by the MPS

We have already seen that the network of blood and lymphatic vessels within the body combined with the MPS provides natural routes for the distribution of nutrients and the clearing of unwanted material. When injected intravenously, particulates are cleared rapidly due to the action of the liver and spleen macrophages and this site-specific, but passive, mechanism of clearance is a feature of the immune system. After macrophage uptake, the drug carrier will be transported to lysosomes and the drug can be released upon breakdown of the carrier. Consequently, this mechanism can be used to target these cells and therapeutically can be used for:

- the treatment of macrophage intracellular microbial, viral or bacterial disease (e.g. visceral leishmaniasis)
- the treatment of lysosomal enzyme deficiencies (e.g. Gaucher's disease, caused by a deficiency of the enzyme glucosylceramidase).

Tip

Visceral leishmaniasis (also known as black fever) is a *Leishmania* parasite infection. The parasite accumulates in the liver, spleen and bone marrow of the host. Symptoms include fever, weight loss, anaemia and swelling of the liver and spleen. Treatment includes the use of AmBisome, Abelcet and Amphocil, which are all formulations of amphotericin B. These are discussed in detail in Chapter 8.

If passively targeting specific lymph nodes, interstitial injection may be a preferred option. The size and surface characteristics of the particles injected by this route again control their residence time at the target site, with particles less than 100 nm rapidly leaking into the blood capillaries.

Local physiological conditions

In addition to exploiting the action of the MPS, passive targeting can take place as a result of the local conditions in the body. The local pH or presence of specific enzymes within a target organ can also be used to facilitate the release of the active drug from its carrier system specifically at these sites. For example, elevated enzyme levels at a target site can be used to release the active drug selectively from its prodrug or carrier system. Enzymes such as alkaline phosphatase and plasmin are known to have increased levels at tumour sites. This is discussed in more detail in Chapter 8.

Enhanced permeability and retention (EPR) effect

As mentioned in the section on escape from the systemic circulation, the integrity of the endothelial barrier at sites of inflammation or tumours is often disrupted by the presence of endothelial fenestrations as large as 200–300 nm. The change in the tumour endothelial barrier is a result of angiogenesis occurring during tumour growth which results in defective hypervasculature and a deficient lymphatic drainage system. This modified permeability of the endothelium resulting from pathological conditions can be exploited in drug-targeting strategies to allow the escape of the drug carrier from the central circulation. This phenomenon is called the enhanced permeability and retention, or EPR, effect.

The EPR effect can be exploited to target drug carriers passively to a site where the vasculature is leaky and gaps in the endothelium are present, such as sites of inflammation or certain tumour sites. However, for this to take effect, the delivery system should be designed to avoid their recognition and clearance by the MPS (via modification of its surface characteristics and size; as already discussed) such that the circulation time in the blood compartment is long enough to allow the carrier to accumulate at the tumour site and release the drug. Targeting via the EPR effect is driven by the plasma concentration of the delivery system (Figure 7.4).

Tip

Angiogenesis is the growth of new capillary blood vessels in the body. It is an important process necessary for the repair or regeneration of tissue during wound healing.

The hyperpermeability of the tumour vasculature is a key feature controlling the targeting of liposomes (e.g. Caelyx/Doxil) and polymer-based (e.g. Oncaspar) cancer therapies. Due to the leaky vasculature of the tumour site, after intravenous injection these drug carriers can either selectively move into the tumour tissue directly,

Figure 7.4 Representation of the enhanced permeability of the endothelial barrier at sites of inflammation and tumours which can facilitate escape from the circulation.

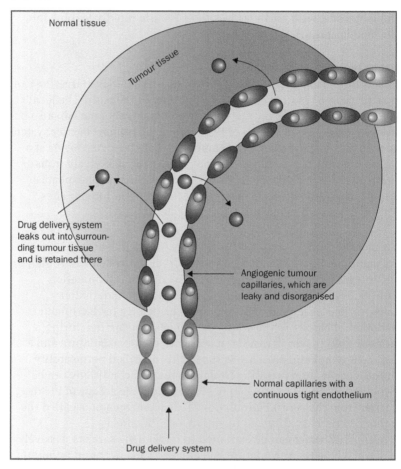

Normal tissue

Tumour tissue

Drug delivery system leaks out into surrounding tumour tissue and is retained there

Angiogenic tumour capillaries, which are leaky and disorganised

Normal capillaries with a continuous tight endothelium

Drug delivery system

Tip

Caelyx is a formulation of doxorubicin encapsulated within liposomes. Oncaspar is a polymer conjugated enzyme (asparaginase). These are discussed in detail in Chapter 8.

KeyPoint

- Active targeting is based on ligand–receptor binding and takes advantage of elevated levels of such receptors at a target site.

or the particulate carrier system can become trapped in the tumour vasculature and release its drug load locally, where again due to the leaky vasculature it can reach the tumour tissue. As the tumour tissue generally lacks effective lymphatic drainage, this further promotes the retention and accumulation of the drug and delivery system.

Active targeting

With active targeting we are relying on the interactions between a targeting moiety and a corresponding receptor to facilitate the targeting of a carrier to a specific cell. These targeting groups are generally covalently, rather than non-covalently, attached to the drug or the surface of the carrier. There are various molecules/receptors that can be used to facilitate active targeting. However it is important to remember that if active targeting is to be effective, the carrier system should be designed to avoid the passive targeting route, particularly the phagocytes of the MPS.

Targeting via folate receptors

Folate can be used as a targeting mechanism for drug delivery. Folate receptors, which bind the vitamin folic acid, are generally found in low levels in most tissues but these receptors are overexpressed in tumour tissues. After receptor binding, folate is rapidly taken up into the cell by endocytosis. This offers an opportunity to target such malignant tissues. The folate receptor is particularly well suited for tumour-targeted drug delivery because the receptor is up-regulated in many human cancers, and receptor density appears to increase as the stage/grade of the cancer progresses.

Antibodies – antigen targeting

Antibodies are circulating plasma proteins which are produced by the adaptive immune system and bind to specific target molecules, referred to as antigens. These antigens are generally proteins or polysaccharides. Antigens can be present on a range of cells such as tumour cells or invading pathogens such as bacteria, viruses and other microorganisms. By exploiting this characteristic, antibodies can be used as drugs in their own right and actively to target a range of cells, either by directly conjugating a drug to the antibody or by using the antibody as the targeting group for drug carriers. Antibodies as targeting devices and carriers are discussed in more detail in Chapter 8.

Lectin – glycoprotein targeting

Lectins are proteins which are capable of recognising and specifically binding to glycoproteins. Glycoproteins are located on the surface of microbial cells and as such can be used to target invading pathogens. Lectins are also overexpressed on the surface of many tumour cells and as such can also be used for targeting via the use of a glycoprotein as the targeting moiety.

Physical targeting

The preferential distribution of a delivery system to a target site can also be controlled physically by means such as magnetically controlled drug delivery. This method is based on binding drugs to magnetic compounds and concentrating the drug in the target area using magnetic fields. These systems can target locations but not to the accuracy of given cell types. Magnetically controlled drug delivery systems have been tested in patients; however no formulations are available for clinical application.

Another way of delivering a drug to its target of action is to implant a pump with programmable drug feed. The Synchromed II spasticity pump is an example of these systems. The drug baclofen is pumped with a catheter into the spinal marrow fluid and acts directly at the nervous system. The pump is programmed depending on the required amount of drug and a refill of the pump is only necessary every few months.

KeyPoints

- Many drugs require cytosolic delivery because their target is located within the cell.
- Macromolecules and particulates enter cells by phagocytosis and receptor-mediated endocytosis.
- Intracellular targets include the nucleus and mitochondria.

Tip

There are various receptors that can mediate endosomal uptake, including galactose receptors on the surface of hepatocytes and macrophages and transferrin receptors on the endothelia of the blood–brain barrier. Targeting of these receptors can be exploited in active targeting strategies.

Cellular uptake and intracellular routing of the drug

Depending on the final target of a drug, the delivery system may need to cross cellular and possibly intracellular membranes. Therefore additional barriers will also be presented (e.g. transcellular or paracellular transport, efflux; Chapter 1).

There are various pathways to enter a cell. Small drugs can enter by diffusion across the cell membrane by virtue of a concentration gradient. Specific carrier proteins in cell membranes can also transport drugs into cells. This transport process can operate against a concentration gradient. However, generally macromolecules and particulate delivery systems are too large to enter by such means.

All eukaryotic cells take up macromolecules through endocytosis, the mechanism by which large or polar substances are engulfed by the cell membrane and entrapped in an intracellular vesicle within the cell.

There are various types of endocytosis (Figure 7.5):

- Phagocytosis – where particulates are engulfed
- Pinocytosis – where fluids are taken up
- Receptor-mediated endocytosis – this involves active binding of a ligand to a membrane-bound receptor. These receptors are generally associated with a cytosolic fibrous protein, clarathin, and binding to these receptors triggers the cytoplasm to fold inwards to form clarathin-coated pits. This process is saturable.

After invagination of the cell membrane and vesicle formation (e.g. phagosomes and endosomes), these vesicles fuse with one or more lysosomes, which results in a drop in pH and digestion of the contents by various enzymes.

Figure 7.5 Endocytotic pathways for drug entry into a cell.

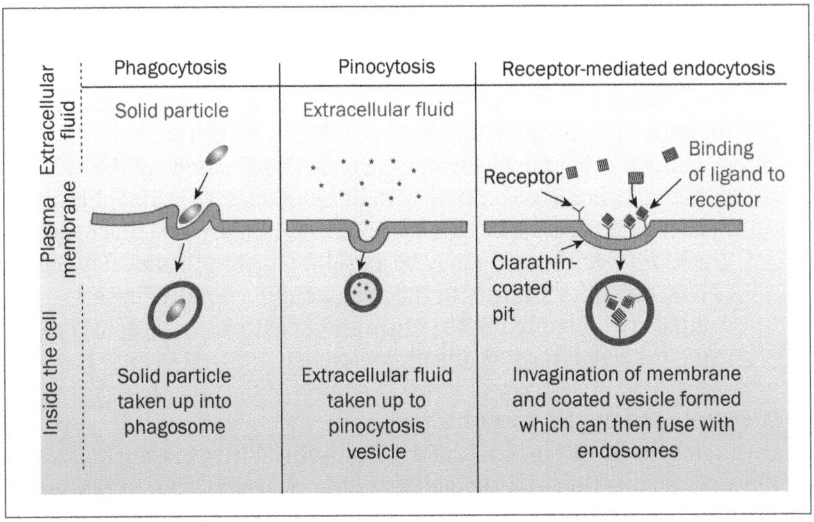

Cytoplasmic delivery

The majority of drugs exert their action within the cytoplasm of the cell where their target enzymes are located. The drug therefore must escape the endosomal vesicles. Several strategies have been investigated to facilitate and enhance the release from the endosomal compartment, including the use of delivery systems that can destabilise the endosomal membrane at low pH and inclusion of peptides or proteins in the delivery system that can fuse with the endosomal membrane. This latter mechanism is also used by several viruses to promote escape from the endosome into the cytosol. Once in the cytosol there are a range of sites that a drug may need to target:

- Nuclear targeting: macromolecules frequently enter and exit the nucleus during normal cell function, but access to the nucleus is tightly controlled by a double membrane that encloses the entire organelle. If the drug requires entry within the nucleus to have its therapeutic action, nuclear targeting is also required. This is the case for intercalating agents or in gene therapy where DNA is the target. Entry into the nucleus takes place via pores in the nuclear membrane. These pores are a complex of about 100 proteins that are arranged into a tunnel that penetrates the nuclear bilayer. Small molecules can pass through these pores via passive diffusion whilst larger molecules (> 45 kDa) must have a specific targeting signal, known as a nuclear localisation signal, which can bind to specific proteins (known as importins) on the nuclear envelope and which mediate transport in and out of the nucleus.

■ Mitochondrial targeting: the mitochondria within cells synthesise adenosine triphosphate and help control cell metabolism, intracellular calcium levels and apoptosis. Within the mitochondria there is a small genome that codes for 13 hydrophobic proteins, all involved in electron transfer. Diseases related to mitochondrial function are a result of damage to this DNA and changes in the proteins involved in electron transport. Dysfunctions of the mitochondria are associated with diseases such as schizophrenia, Alzheimer's disease, Parkinson's disease, epilepsy and diabetes. Therefore mitochondria may be a useful target in the development of new therapies. Similar to the nucleus, mitochondria have a complex two-membrane structure and targeting can be achieved using mitochondrial localisation proteins.

Drug release at the target site

Ultimately at the target site the drug must be able to exert its physiological action and the ability of the carrier system to release the drug at the target site is important to ensure sufficiently high drug concentrations at the target. The mechanism of release depends on the carrier system employed and it needs to be at a rate that ensures drug accumulation at the target site. However, to avoid free drug reaching non-target sites, it is important that the drug remains associated with the carrier during transit in the circulation. Early release will result in low concentrations of the drug at the target site and non-specific distribution. Conversely, the rate of elimination of any free drug released into the systemic circulation should ideally be rapid so as to maintain a high target:non-target drug concentration ratio.

Summary

For effective targeting the target must be well defined with unique properties and easy to reach. The drug must also be effective at the site, and the delivery system should be formulated such that it allows effective targeting to the desired site and release of the active drug at the appropriate concentration and duration. The range of delivery systems that are available and their mechanism of drug release will be considered in Chapter 8.

Self-assessment

After having read this chapter you should be able to:
■ describe the advantages of using drug-targeting systems
■ identify key characteristics of an effective drug delivery system
■ give examples of possible targets for drug delivery
■ discuss the barriers to drug delivery
■ discuss how drug carriers are eliminated from the body

- discuss how to design a carrier system to avoid opsonisation and MPS recognition
- describe how drugs are passively targeted in the body
- discuss the physicochemical properties of the carrier
- describe how the EPR effect can enhance tumour targeting
- compare and contrast passive and active targeting strategies
- describe how drug delivery systems can enter cells and reach intracellular targets.

Questions

1. **Indicate which one of the following statements is not correct:**
a. An ideal drug-targeting system should be non-toxic and therapeutically acceptable.
b. An ideal drug-targeting system should specifically target the drug to the physiological target.
c. An ideal drug-targeting system should release the drug in a controlled fashion during transit to the target site.
d. In an ideal drug-targeting system the drug must be able to access the target site.
e. In an ideal drug-targeting system the drug should be retained at the site.

2. **Indicate which one of the following statements is not correct:**
a. There are various sites and levels to which one can target a drug, including specific organs, tissues, invading organisms, specific cells, cytosolic targets and subcellular compartments.
b. The physicochemical nature of a drug carrier system can dictate the fate and distribution of the drug.
c. To reach the targets one can either chemically modify the drug using a prodrug approach or use a carrier system.
d. Soluble carrier systems include natural and synthetic water-soluble polymers and antibodies. With these systems the drug is conjugated to the carrier.
e. Particulate carrier systems include liposomes, microspheres and nanoparticles. With these systems the drug has to be surface-bound to the carrier.

3. **Indicate which one of the following statements is not correct:**
a. Depending on the physiology of the target, some drug-targeting systems may naturally accumulate at the target site (known as passive targeting).
b. Some drug-targeting systems may be actively targeted to a site using a target-specific recognition component.
c. Drug-targeting systems can be understood as 'homing devices' which purposely search out the target.
d. Addition of galactose to a carrier system can promote targeting of galactose receptors on the surface of liver parenchymal cells.

4.   Indicate which one of the following statements is not correct:

a.   To reach internal organs a drug must leave the central circulation by crossing the endothelium.

b.   Drug carrier systems tend to have similar biodistribution profiles to the parent drug.

c.   Current drug-targeting systems are generally developed for administration via the parenteral route.

d.   Unlike free drugs, drug carrier systems are generally too large to be eliminated by the kidney.

e.   A major barrier that drug delivery systems must be able to overcome in the systemic circulation is the reticuloendothelial system.

5.   Indicate which one of the following statements is not correct:

a.   The cells of the reticuloendothelial system originate from the bone marrow.

b.   The main function of the phagocytic cells of the reticuloendothelial system is to eliminate and remove foreign material, including bacteria and proteins.

c.   The phagocytic cells of the reticuloendothelial system are involved in antigen processing and presentation as part of the immune response.

d.   Macrophages in the lymph nodes are termed Kupffer cells.

e.   When injected intravenously, particles can be quickly cleared from the circulation by the liver and spleen macrophages of the reticuloendothelial system.

6.   Indicate which one of the following statements is not correct:

a.   Opsonisation is a process in which the surface of a particle or pathogen is coated by molecules known as opsonins.

b.   Blood opsonic factors include fibronection, antibodies and complement proteins.

c.   Opsonisation of foreign particles is a method of marking the particulates for easier recognition and destruction by reticuloendothelial system phagocytes.

d.   Phagocytes carry surface receptors that bind to the opsonins.

e.   Antibodies (in particular immunoglobulin (IgG) also act as opsonins by binding to sites through their Fc region, leaving the Fab region free.

7.   Indicate which one of the following statements is not correct:

a.   Charged particles tend to remain longer in circulation compared to their neutral counterparts.

b.   Particles of 1–2 µm are effectively cleared by phagocytosis, whereas particulates in the range of 2–20 µm tend to become trapped in the lung capillaries.

c.   Adding a hydrophilic coat to a carrier system reduces protein adsorption and opsonisation, thus suppressing macrophage recognition.

d. Poly(ethyleneglycol) coating is commonly used as a hydrophilic coat for a carrier system.

8. **Indicate which one of the following statements is not correct:**
a. A targeted drug delivery system generally needs to leave the vasculature before it can reach its target.
b. The structure of the blood capillary wall varies in different organs and tissues.
c. Sinusoidal blood capillary walls have gaps of up to 1.5 µm between them and the basement membrane is absent.
d. Fenestrated blood capillary walls have gaps of 20–80 nm between the endothelial cells.
e. Continuous blood capillary walls are widely distributed in the body. They have tight junctions between the endothelial cells and a continuous basement membrane.

9. **Indicate which one of the following statements is not correct:**
a. Passive targeting uses targeting groups such as antibodies to bind to specific receptors on cells.
b. After macrophage uptake, a drug carrier will be transported to lysosomes and the drug can be released upon breakdown of the carrier.
c. The mechanism described in **b** can be used to target macrophages for the treatment of macrophage intracellular microbial, viral or bacterial diseases.
d. The mechanism described in **b** can be used to target macrophages for the treatment of lysosomal enzyme deficiencies.

10. **Indicate which one of the following statements is not correct:**
a. Increased permeability of the endothelium due to pathological conditions can be exploited to allow the escape of the drug carrier from the central circulation.
b. The phenomenon described in **a** is called the enhanced permeability and retention (EPR) effect.
c. Due to the leaky vasculature of the tumour site, after intravenous injection particulate carrier systems can become trapped in the tumour vasculature.
d. Tumour tissue generally lacks effective lymphatic drainage.
e. Targeting via the EPR effect is driven by active targeting moieties on the drug delivery system.

11. **Indicate which one of the following statements is not correct.**
a. For active targeting to be effective, the carrier system should be designed to avoid the passive targeting route, particularly the phagocytes of the reticuloendothelial system.
b. For active targeting, targeting groups are generally non-covalently, rather than covalently, attached to the drug or the surface of the carrier.

c. Folate can be used as a targeting moiety for active targeting because the folate receptor is up-regulated in many human cancers.

d. Antibodies can be used as drugs in their own right and to target a range of cells actively.

e. Lectins are overexpressed on the surface of many tumour cells and as such can be used for targeting with glycoproteins as the targeting moiety.

12. Indicate which one of the following statements is not correct.

a. Small drugs can enter cells by diffusion across the cell membrane.

b. Some drugs are actively transported into cells by specific carrier proteins in cell membranes.

c. Receptor-mediated endocytosis is a mechanism for particulate uptake into cells and involves active binding of a ligand to a membrane-bound receptor.

d. Phagocytosis is a process in which fluids are taken up into the cell.

e. Large molecules (> 45 kDa) must have a specific targeting signal known as a nuclear localisation signal which can bind to specific proteins (known as importins) on the nuclear envelope to enter the nucleus.

Further reading

Hillery A *et al.* (2001) *Drug Delivery and Targeting for Pharmacists and Pharmaceutical Scientists.* London: Taylor and Francis.

Kumar V, Banker GS (2002) Target-oriented drug delivery systems. In: Banker GS, Rhodes CT (eds) *Modern Pharmaceutics*, 4th edn. London: Informa Healthcare.

Moghimi SM *et al.* Nanomedicine: current status and future prospects. *FASEB J* 19:2005; 311–330.

Petrak K Essential properties of drug-targeting delivery systems. *Drug Disc Today* 10:2005; 1667–1673.

Wilson CG, Washington N (1989) *Physiological Pharmaceutics*. Chichester: Ellis Horwood.

chapter 8

Carriers for drug targeting

Overview

In this chapter we will:

- differentiate and discuss the various options which can be used to promote site-directed drug targeting
- discuss how prodrugs can be designed to give targeted drug delivery
- discuss the use of antibodies as actively targeted drugs, and their use in actively targeting carrier systems
- discuss how polymer conjugates can improve the delivery of proteins and drugs and be designed to exploit the enhanced permeability and retention (EPR) effect
- describe the various nanoparticulates and colloidal systems used for drug targeting, including:
- dendrimers
- nanoparticles
- micelles
- liposomes
- microspheres
- discuss how these systems can be designed for passive and active targeting and review various examples of products used clinically.

Options for drug targeting systems

As noted in Chapter 7, drug targeting can be achieved through both passive and active targeting, with passive targeting being based on the distribution of the carrier via:

- the actions of the mononuclear phagocyte system (MPS)
- the EPR effect.

By contrast active targeting requires the use of targeting groups to bind to specific receptors or ligands on cells, with antibody targeting being the main strategy used clinically. To exploit these targeting

KeyPoints

- Drugs can be targeted passively or actively.
- To exploit and control these targeting options the drug can be modified, conjugated to a carrier or loaded on to a delivery system.
- There is a range of delivery systems available from macromolecules up to particulate systems.

mechanisms and achieve site-specific drug targeting there are a range of delivery systems that can be used. These can be categorised generally into three main strategies:

1. Modification of the drug at the molecular level: using prodrug systems.

2. Macromolecular targeting carriers: using soluble drug carriers, including antibody carriers and polymeric conjugates.
3. Colloidal/particulate carrier systems: these can include dendrimers, nanoparticles, micelles, emulsions, liposomes and their various derivatives, and microspheres.

However the distinction between these three categories is somewhat arbitrary with fuzzy boundaries: many macromolecular targeting systems fall within the colloidal (nanometre) size range and particulate systems may sometimes be in the micrometre size range. The choice of delivery systems depends on a variety of factors, including:

- the physicochemical characteristics of the drug
- the physiology and location of the target site
- the mechanism of targeting
- the dose required
- the route of administration.

Considering the pharmacokinetics of a drug, association of a drug with any of the delivery systems discussed within this chapter will have dramatic effects, changing its absorption, volume of distribution, clearance and metabolism. Generally, with the exception of prodrugs, the systems discussed are formulated for intravenous injection and often used for the delivery of drugs with severe side-effect profiles. Thus the primary aim of these carriers is to reduce acute toxicity by enhancing targeting. Some of these systems are also used clinically for other administration routes, e.g. for oral administration of low-solubility drugs, and have been considered for these applications in previous chapters.

Modification of the drug to promote targeting – prodrugs

Prodrugs have already been defined as compounds which undergo biotransformation either by a chemical or enzymatic reaction before exhibiting a biological response. In the context of drug targeting, a variety of mechanisms can be used to achieve this aim by using prodrugs. However the key prerequisites for a prodrug are that it should be readily taken up and transported to the target site. At the target site there should be

Tips

The various delivery systems are sometimes classified by size; however this is not ideal given that some molecules are within the nanometre size range and could be classified as macromolecules, nanoparticles or colloidal delivery systems.

Examples of approximate sizes are:

- A water molecule: 0.16 nm
- A spherical 'buckyball' C_{60} fullerene: 0.73 nm
- A haemoglobulin molecule: 6.4 nm
- An antibody: 7.5 nm
- Micelles: 5–50 nm
- Dendrimers: 1–100 nm
- Nanoparticles: 1–100 nm
- Liposomes: >30 nm up to several micrometres.

KeyPoint

- Prodrugs can be designed to release the active drug at specific sites by exploiting differences in the local environment at the site of action, such as elevated enzyme levels.

selective cleavage of the prodrug and activation of the drug. Finally, once generated, the active drug should be retained at the site of action.

Site-specific localisation

We have already seen how prodrugs can be used to enhance the solubility and absorption of drugs (Chapters 2 and 3 respectively). Prodrugs can also be formulated to promote site-specific localisation by exploiting the physicochemical properties of the prodrug and the activated form to retain high drug concentrations at the site of action. For example, L-dopa, an amino acid prodrug of dopamine, is actively transported across the blood–brain barrier and metabolised to dopamine in the brain (Figure 8.1). Dopamine is hydrophilic and protonated at body pH and has good water solubility. However its low lipid solubility results in poor blood–brain

Tip

Levodopa is used in the treatment of Parkinson's disease, which involves the progressive degeneration of neurons in certain regions of the brain, which in turn leads to a deficiency of the neurotransmitter dopamine. Current drug therapy improves patient quality of life but does not prevent disease progression.

Figure 8.1 L-Dopa transformation into dopamine, which becomes trapped within the brain. CNS, central nervous system; BBB, blood–brain barrier.

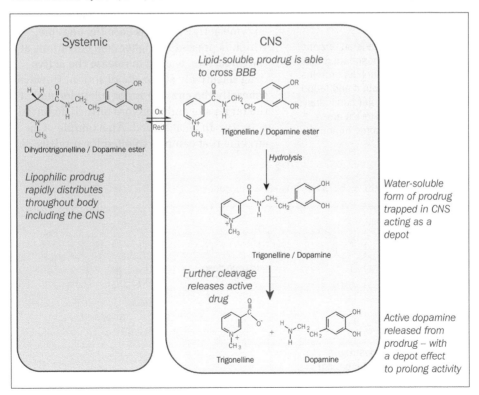

barrier transport and subsequently it is not absorbed into the brain. The amino acid functional group in the prodrug enhances the transport of the prodrug across the blood–brain barrier, and then undergoes activation to dopamine via dopa decarboxylase. The water-soluble dopamine becomes trapped in the central nervous system due to its physical attributes, hindering transport back across the blood–brain barrier. However L-dopa is converted to dopamine both in the brain and in the peripheral tissues, resulting in unwanted side-effects. This problem can be limited by the co-administration of carbidopa, a decarboxylase inhibitor, which inhibits conversion of L-dopa in the circulation and peripheral tissue. Carbidopa does not cross the blood–brain barrier and therefore the conversion of L-dopa to dopamine within the brain is unaffected.

Tip

The endothelial cells of capillaries in the brain are different from those found in peripheral tissues as the cells are sealed together with tight junctions and no transcellular drug transport occurs. Lipid-soluble molecules such as ethanol and caffeine can easily cross the cell membrane and gain access to the brain.

Site-specific activation of prodrugs

Prodrugs can also be designed to release their active drug at a specific site of action by exploiting a particular target site pathophysiology such as an enhanced enzyme activity. In this case the enzyme, which is present in higher concentrations at the target site, is used to release the active drug selectively at the site of action. However generally the enzyme is not solely located at the target site and therefore only differential activity can be achieved. An example of an enzyme that can be exploited for prodrug

Tip

Alkaline phosphate is an enzyme which removes phosphate groups from molecules such as proteins. It is membrane-bound and found in the liver, bone, gut and kidney; however elevated levels are associated with some tumours.

Figure 8.2 Stilboestrol diphosphate breakdown to stilboestrol.

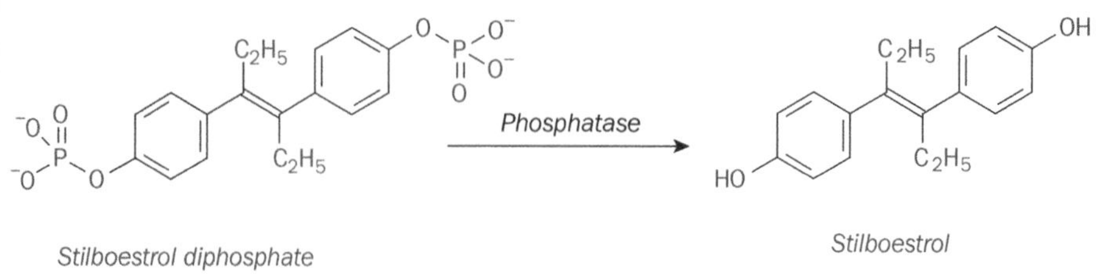

Stilboestrol diphosphate

Synthetic oestrogen
used in prostatic cancer

Phosphatase

Stilboestrol

activation is alkaline phosphatase which is present at significantly higher levels in tumour sites. The prodrug stilboestrol diphosphate, a synthetic oestrogen used in the treatment of prostatic cancer, is designed to be cleaved by phosphatase to the active form of the drug, stilboestrol (Figure 8.2).

Limitations of using prodrugs for drug targeting

When considering the application of prodrugs for site-directed drug delivery the pharmacokinetics of both the prodrug and active drug must be considered. The prodrug must have good access to the target organ and pharmacological site of action, and the active drug must show a good retention at that site. Consideration should also be given to the possibility of toxicity associated with the prodrug and its metabolites. Finally the distribution, relative activity and specificity of the enzyme responsible for prodrug activation must be known.

Soluble macromolecular drug carriers to promote targeting

The main benefit of using a drug carrier system to facilitate drug targeting is that the distribution of drugs in the body can be dictated by the carrier system rather than the physicochemical characteristics of the drug. However, the conjugation of a drug to a carrier system can also change the carrier properties depending on the overall contribution of each component to the overall characteristics of the conjugate. There are a range of options for drug carriers which span from soluble macromolecules to larger particulate carriers.

> **KeyPoints**
>
> - Soluble macromolecular carriers, including antibodies, polymers and proteins, can be used to support site-directed drug targeting.
> - The small size of these carriers compared to particulate systems facilitates their movement out of the systemic circulation; however they can carry less drug.

Soluble drug carriers have an advantage over particulate carriers in their greater ability to extravasate and escape from the systemic circulation. Their plasma half-life is based on their molecular weight, ionic nature, configuration and interaction with biological components in circulation. Relative to particulate drug delivery systems, the main limitation of these systems is their low drug-carrying capacity. The covalent attachment of the drug to the carrier may also inhibit the activity of the drug. There are various macromolecules that can be used as carriers, including antibodies and their fragments, synthetic polymers, proteins and polysaccharides. In all cases, these carriers should be:

- non-toxic
- non-immunogenic
- suitable for repeated administration.

KeyPoints

- Antibodies are large proteins produced by B cells.
- They can target antigens and so can be used as targeted drugs in their own right or as targeting groups which are conjugated to other drugs or carrier systems.
- Whilst there are several classes of antibodies, most clinically approved products are based on immunoglobulin (IgG) antibodies.

Antibodies as drugs and delivery systems

Antibodies (also known as immunoglobulins) are large, complex protein macromolecules produced by B cells to recognise and specifically target foreign materials, known as antigens. This allows for the use of antibodies actively to target specific cell types. Antibodies can be used as drugs in their own right or as a targeting group attached to a drug or carrier system. As targeting groups, antibodies have the advantage of high specificity, due to their antigen recognition and targeting capability. However, due to their protein nature, antibodies can be subject to a range of purity and instability issues similar to those outlined for protein carriers.

There are several classes of antibodies produced in the human body and the five main types are IgG, IgA, IgM, IgE and IgD. Of these, IgG is the most abundant and most of the currently approved antibody-based drugs are of the IgG class. The basic structure of an IgG antibody molecule comprises two identical heavy chains (50 kDa molecular weight) and two light chains (23 kDa molecular weight) (Figure 8.3). These chains are held together by non-covalent interactions and disulfide bonds. The specificity of a given antibody is determined by the amino acid sequence located at the end of its so-called Fab region (where 'F' stands for fragment and 'ab' stands for antigen binding).

Figure 8.3 Immunoglobulin G (IgG) antibody.

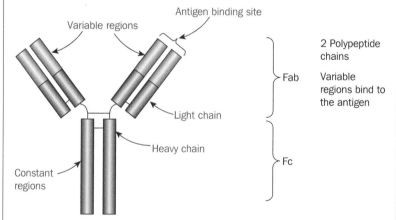

Polyclonal antibody drug therapies

Polyclonal antibodies were the first therapeutic antibody systems available. Whilst not an obvious drug targeting system, polyclonal antibodies are derived from different B cells responding against an antigen, so they are a mixture of antibodies targeted against different epitopes of a specific antigen. Polyclonal antibodies are used to induce passive immunisation against infectious diseases and other harmful agents. They may be categorised into several groups based on their target specificities with antibodies raised against specific microbial or viral pathogens and microbial toxins, and antibodies raised against snake/spider venoms (antivenoms). Polyclonal antibodies can be given in the form of antisera which are sterile preparations containing immunoglobulins obtained from the serum of immunised animals by purification. Immunoglobulins can also be prepared from human plasma or serum, taken from blood donors. They are usually administered intravenously and can be used both prophylactically (e.g. administration of an antisnake toxin antibody prior to travelling) or therapeutically (e.g. antivenom antibody after a snake bite). Whilst these systems are not examples of drug delivery systems they can be classed as examples of targeted drug therapies in a wider context.

> ### KeyPoints
>
> - Polyclonal antibodies are a mixture of antibodies targeted to a specific antigen.
> - They can induce passive immunisation and can be used prophylactically or therapeutically.

Polyclonal antibody therapies

- *Botulinum Antitoxin (Ph Eur) and Botulism Antitoxin (USP 25).* These are sterile preparations containing specific antitoxic antibodies which can target and neutralise the toxins formed by *Clostridium botulinum*. These are used in the postexposure prophylaxis and treatment of botulism. Botulism is caused by the exotoxin of *C. botulinum*, a spore-forming, Gram-positive anaerobic microorganism found in soil and mud. Normally the disease results from eating contaminated food, but it may also develop from infected wounds. Infant botulism is of increasing concern.

- *Human hepatitis B immunoglobulins.* These are used for passive immunisation of people potentially exposed to the hepatitis B virus. They are not appropriate for treatment. Active immunisation with hepatitis B vaccine should always be commenced in conjunction with administration of hepatitis B immunoglobulins in patients exposed to the virus.

Monoclonal antibody drug therapies

Monoclonal antibodies are produced from a single B-cell hybridoma cell line using hybridoma technology. In contrast to polyclonal antibodies, monoclonal antibodies are produced by a single cloned

B-cell line, and single specificity antibodies can be produced. Due to their targeting properties, monoclonal antibodies can be used as:

- 'Naked' monoclonal antibodies: these have no drug or radioactive material attached to them.
- Conjugated monoclonal antibodies: monoclonal antibodies joined to a chemotherapeutic drug, radioactive substance or toxin.

In both cases their ability to recognise a given antigen allows them to bind to particular proteins/antigens on a cell surface. The formation of such complexes can result in the receptor action being down-regulated and/or blocked or it may stimulate the recognition and destruction of cells by the host immune system (Figure 8.4).

As therapeutic agents, there are several monoclonal antibody-based products clinically used which have been developed to target a range of sites (Table 8.1). Key advances in the production of monoclonal antibodies, including the improved ability to produce appropriate quantities of pure antibodies and, more importantly, the ability to prepare humanised antibodies, have supported their increased application. Prior to this, the use of murine-based antibody therapeutics (e.g. OKT-3, muromonab-CD3, approved for use within the USA) resulted in antibody therapies generally being limited to acute, single treatments such as tissue rejection after a kidney transplant. The use of murine antibodies often results in the patient's immune system inducing human antimouse antibodies that can lead to lack of efficacy, rapid clearance of the antibody and adverse reactions to the antibody. Recombinant technologies have allowed the production of fewer immunogenic monoclonal antibodies: chimeric antibodies (e.g. rituximab) are composed of murine variable regions fused with human constant

KeyPoints

- Monoclonal antibodies are produced from a single B-cell hybridoma cell line.
- They can be used as targeting drugs or as a targeting carrier system.
- There are several antibody products clinically available.

Tip

B-cell hybridoma cells are created from the fusion of a B cell with a cancer cell such as myeloma or lymphoma cells. Due to this fusion, the cells proliferate and produce a continuous supply of a specific monoclonal antibody.

Figure 8.4 Action of monoclonal antibodies as drug therapies.

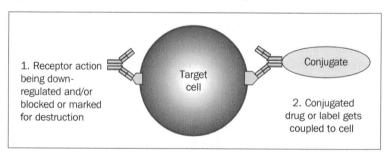

1. Receptor action being down-regulated and/or blocked or marked for destruction

Target cell

Conjugate

2. Conjugated drug or label gets coupled to cell

Table 8.1 Licensed monoclonal antibodies

Generic name	Trade name	Type of antibody	Target	Indications*
Abciximab	ReoPro	Chimeric	Platelet glycoprotein IIb/IIIa	Prevention of cardiac complications in patients scheduled for percutaneous coronary intervention
Adalimumab	Humira	Human	TNF-alpha	Severe Crohn's disease, ankylosing spondylitis, psoriatic arthritis, rheumatoid arthritis
Bevacizumab	Avastin	Humanised	Vascular endothelial growth factor	Treatment of metastatic colorectal cancer and unresectable advanced metastatic or recurrent non-small-cell lung cancer
Palivizumab	Synagis	Humanised	F protein of RSV	Prevention of serious lower respiratory tract disease caused by RSV in children
Rituximab	Mabthera	Chimeric	CD20	Follicular lymphoma and non-Hodgkin's lymphoma. Also used in the treatment of rheumatoid arthritis
Trastuzumab	Herceptin	Humanised	HER2 growth receptor	Early breast cancer which overexpresses HER2

* Indications based on *British National Formulary* 55 (2008) London: BMJ Publishing/RPS Publishing.
TNF, tumour necrosis factor; RSV, respiratory syncytial virus; HER2, human epidermal growth factor receptor-2.

regions, whereas humanised antibodies (e.g. trastuzumab) are produced by grafting murine hypervariable amino acid domains into human antibodies. Complete human monoclonal antibody constructs can now also be produced (e.g. adalimumab) due to developments in phage display technology and the availability of transgenic mice (Figure 8.5).

Tip

Humira (adalimumab) was the first phage display antibody, produced in 2002 by Cambridge Antibody Technology.

Antibody therapies

- *Mabthera (rituximab).* Mabthera antibodies bind to the CD20 protein. This can be used in the treatment of non-Hodgkin's lymphoma where B cells overexpress the CD20 protein on their surface. It is thought that binding of monoclonal antibodies to these B cells results in their targeted destruction either through the Fc region of the antibody activating complement and/or the binding of the antibody to the CD20 protein causing programmed cell death of the B cells.
- *Rimicade (infliximab).* These monoclonal antibodies act as cytokine modulators by binding to tumour necrosis factor-alpha (TNF-alpha), neutralising it and thus limiting its action. TNF-alpha is a cytokine known to play a key role in the pathophysiology of rheumatoid arthritis and other immune inflammatory disorders.

Figure 8.5 Schematic representation of the chimeric antibodies.

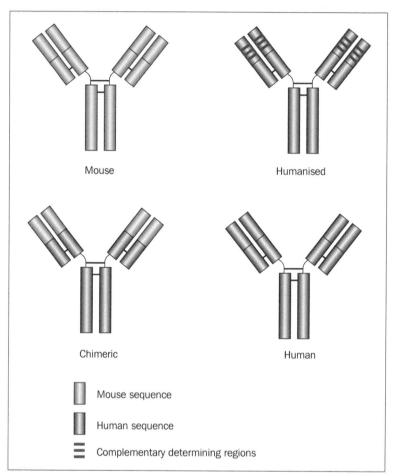

- *Herceptin (trastuzumab).* These antibodies target cells expressing human epidermal growth factor receptor (HER2) protein and therefore can be used to treat persistent, aggressive HER2-driven metastatic cancers. The antibody attaches to HER2 protein receptors on cell surfaces, prevents human epidermal growth factor attaching to the protein, which causes down-regulation of the receptor and limits signals for further cell growth.

Antibody-targeted drug conjugates

In addition to their action as drugs, antibodies can also be used to target drugs and as targeting groups for other drug carriers. Currently there are three antibody conjugates (sometimes referred to as immunoconjugates) used clinically, two of which are radionuclide conjugates:

- ibritumomab tuixetan (Zevalin), which is a murine IgG_1 anti-CD20 antibody conjugated to yttrium 90
- tositumomab (Bexxar), also a mouse anti-CD20 antibody but conjugated to iodine 131. Both are used to target B-cell lymphomas and targeting of the radioisotope results in cell death.

There is also a humanised anti-CD33 antibody–cytotoxin conjugate, gemtuzumab (Mylotarg). By binding to CD33 proteins, gemtuzumab targets leukaemia cells. The cytotoxin delivered is N-acetyl-γ-calicheamicin dimethylhydrazine, a toxic antibiotic. After binding to the CD33 protein, the conjugate enters the cells through the endocytic/lysosomal pathway, the antibody is degraded in the lysosome and the cytotoxin is released into the cytosol, resulting in cell death.

> ## KeyPoints
>
> - Conjugation of drugs or markers to antibodies allows for active drug targeting.
> - Conjugation of radionuclides allows for the targeted delivery of radioisotopes which causes the destruction of the targeted cells.
> - Cytotoxins can also be conjugated to antibodies to promote targeted cell death.

Most antibody conjugates have a relatively poor drug-carrying capacity and have a low drug-to-antibody ratio in the range of 3–10, with higher loading often resulting in reduced antibody-binding activity. Cumulatively this will limit the drug concentration at the site of action. Studies on antibody–carrier–drug conjugates such as antibody–hydroxypropylmethacrylate (HPMA)–doxorubicin have been conducted but this approach is seen to be limited by its increased complexity. Antibody-targeting mechanisms to enhance the specific delivery of colloidal drug delivery systems have also been investigated, e.g. with the development of immunomicelles and immune liposomes. These are discussed in the section below on colloidal and particulate drug delivery systems.

Antibody-directed enzyme prodrug therapy (ADEPT)

Rather than taking advantage of elevated enzyme activities at the target site, antibodies can also be used to target an enzyme specifically to a site of action. Conjugating an enzyme to an antibody allows for the site-specific delivery of the enzyme, which in turn can than act as a drug target (Figure 8.6).

- Firstly, the monoclonal antibody–enzyme conjugate is administered.
- A few hours later a prodrug, which can be enzymatically cleaved by the antibody conjugated enzyme, is given.
- When the prodrug comes into contact with the enzyme at the target site the prodrug is cleaved to its active compound.

This method offers enhanced specificity compared with utilising naturally elevated enzyme activities at the target site since enzymes which are elevated at a target site are usually not solely located at that target site, resulting in only differential activity.

Figure 8.6 Antibody-directed enzyme prodrug therapy (ADEPT) mechanism of action.

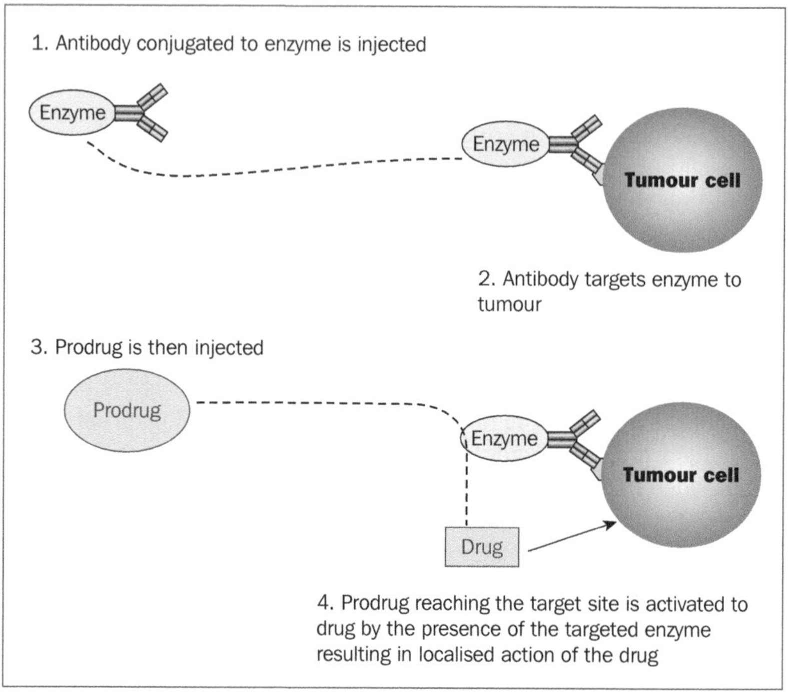

Gene-directed enzyme prodrug therapy (GDEPT)

A further development of enzyme–antibody complexes is the delivery of antibody-coupled genes to the tumour site. In a first step, the gene–antibody complex binds to its target on the tumour cell and is subsequently introduced into the tumour cell. There, the so-called 'suicide genes' code for the prodrug-converting enzyme. In a second step, the non-toxic prodrug is administered and is converted into its active form by the introduced enzyme within the tumour cell, thus allowing site-specific action. Therefore, the main difference between ADEPT and GDEPT is that in GDEPT the prodrug is converted directly in the target cell, leading to higher intracellular concentrations of the drug. Such strategies are currently being investigated in clinical trials for the treatment of prostate cancer.

Antibody fragments

Anitbody fragments, i.e. the antigen-binding Fab fragments, are therapeutically used when binding to the antigen is desired without any activation of effector cells or function (T cells, macrophages, complement binding). In this regard, they display perfect carriers to the desired site of action. They can be used for diagnostic purposes as well as for targeted drug delivery.

Antibody fragments can easily be generated by enzymatic cleavage of full antibodies with papain for Fab fragments and pepsin for F(ab')$_2$ fragments. In the case of F(ab')$_2$ fragments, the binding properties are the same as for full-sized antibodies.

Currently, Fv fragments (only the variable region of Fab fragments) are under investigation as a future drug targeting device. These fragments can be synthesised with genetic engineering methods and their small size enables them to penetrate tissues. Coupled to certain toxins, there is a potential use as targeted cancer therapeutics.

Similar to normal full-sized antibodies, the use of murine fragments presents a major disadvantage since they capture the risk of an immunological response. Repetitive application, therefore, might induce resistance. Examples of murine Fab fragments include the following:

- **Arcitumomab** is a murine Fab fragment coupled to radioactive ^{99m}Tc. It is used as a diagnostic Fab fragment to detect metastases in the body and has no pharmacological effect.
- **Anatumomab mafenatox** in comparison is a target-oriented fusion protein consisting of a murine Fab fragment and the enterotoxin mafenatox of *Staphylococcus aureus*. The antibody fragment targets an overexpressed antigen present on kidney and pancreas tumour cells. Mafenatox is a superantigen which, together with the Fab fragment, is directed towards the tumour cells (tumour-targeted superantigen therapy). Once the antibody fragments bind to the tumour, the attached enterotoxin reveals its superantigen activity and activates cytotoxic T cells that subsequently destroy the tumour cells.

Polymeric conjugates

Synthetic polymers can be custom-made to have defined characteristics such as molecular weight, size and charge, and are generally less immunogenic than naturally derived macromolecules. Synthetic polymers are also generally easier to produce in large quantities at an appropriate quality with higher stability. Unlike the polymers described in Chapter 5 which are used for sustained release, these water-soluble polymer–drug conjugates are intended for parenteral administration and can be designed with passive or active targeting mechanisms.

There are three basic components to polymer–drug conjugate delivery systems: a water-soluble polymer, a linker and the drug (Table 8.2).

KeyPoints

- Drugs can be conjugated to polymers to enhance the site-specific targeting via both passive and active targeting.
- The systems are composed of a polymer backbone and a drug which are conjugated via a linker group. The linker group can be designed to allow for a controlled release of the drug.
- Using poly(ethyleneglycol) (PEG) as the polymer backbone can improve the stability and blood residence time of a drug.
- A targeting group can also be conjugated to the construct.

Table 8.2 Examples of polymer–drug conjugates

Name	Polymer	Linker	Drug
Zinostatin Stimalmer	Syren-maleic anhydride copolymer	Amide	Neocarzinostatin
Oncaspar	m-PEG	Amide	L-Asparaginase
Neulasta	m-PEG	Amide	Granulocyte colony-stimulating factor
PEG-Asys	Branched m-PEG	Amide	Interferon α-2a
PEG-Intron	m-PEG	Carbamate	Interferon α-2b

m-PEG, monomethoxy poly(ethyleneglycol).

Polymer backbone

Soluble synthetic polymers such as PEG, poly(glutamic acid) (PGA) and HPMA copolymers are the most commonly used polymeric-soluble drug carriers. PGA is a biodegradable polymer, whilst both PEG and HPMA are not. Given that polymer clearance from the circulation is dictated by its molecular weight, with clearance rates decreasing with increasing molecular weight up to a threshold of around 45 kDa, non-biodegradable polymers are limited to molecular masses less than 40 kDa to ensure their renal excretion. Above 45 kDa, renal excretion cannot occur and larger polymers are more susceptible to clearance by the mononuclear phagocytic system (MPS).

Water-soluble polymers can also be used to improve the delivery of drugs. In particular, the conjugation of proteins to such polymers can reduce protein immunogenicity and enhance the protein half-life in the circulation and protein stability. The conjugation of PEG to proteins prolongs their half-life by preventing renal elimination and avoiding receptor-mediated protein uptake by the MPS. This allows for a reduced frequency in dosing, which is particularly beneficial for parenterally administered drugs. The PEG content in these systems influences the pharmacokinetic profile of the conjugates. Generally a 1:1 polymer-to-drug ratio is employed with molecular masses of the PEG between 5000 and 40 000 being used in clinical products. PEGylation of proteins, however, may also reduce their biological activity so the conjugation site of the PEG on the protein can be important.

Linker

To the water-soluble polymer backbone the drug can either be directly covalently attached, or more commonly attached via a spacer/linker group (Table 8.2). The use of a spacer group between the polymer and the drug can overcome the problem of the drug's therapeutic action being blocked by the polymer and can also facilitate controlled cleavage of the drug from the carrier, using similar mechanisms to those described for prodrugs. Examples of linkers include amine, carbamate and ester groups which cleave under various conditions. In addition to these components a targeting group (e.g. galactose or an antibody) may also be attached to the polymeric carrier to promote active targeting.

Drug

The majority of these polymer conjugates are used for the delivery of chemotherapy drugs for the treatment of disseminated metastatic diseases. Drugs delivered as polymer conjugates include doxorubicin, paclitaxel and asparaginase. A PEGylated human anti-TNF-alpha Fab fragment is certolizumab pegol. The PEGylation prolongs the blood circulation time of the otherwise unstable Fab fragment. As a result, the circulation of the antibody fragment and its binding to TNF-alpha (inhibiting the function of this inflammatory cytokine) is prolonged. Certolizumab pegol is used for the treatment of rheumatoid arthritis and Crohn's disease.

Overall these polymer–drug conjugate systems are generally below 100 nm in size and can also be seen as a new chemical entity in their own right, similar to prodrugs, rather than as a drug delivery system.

Targeting of polymer-based carrier systems

In addition to improving the stability of proteins, polymer conjugates can enhance targeting of drugs and proteins. Polymer-based cancer therapies can be passively targeted to tumour sites due to the EPR effect (Chapter 7). After intravenous administration, the conjugate escapes the circulation through the leaky tumour

Tip

Lysosomes are intracellular organelles with an acidic interior and contain digestive enzymes. Their role is to digest material taken up by phagocytosis and endocytosis by fusing with the vacuoles formed after phagocytosis or endocytosis.

vasculature. Therefore the extent of EPR-mediated targeting to tumour sites depends on the plasma concentration of the polymer conjugate. The fact that these carrier systems are soluble means that these systems can be taken up into cells by endocytosis or pinocytosis depending on their size. When the carrier reaches the lysosomes, the drug can be released from the carrier through the degradation of the polymeric carrier and/or the spacer group by the action of enzymes or the low-pH conditions present in the lysosome. The free drug may then be released from the lysosome, possibly by diffusion through the lysosome membrane. However the lysosomal membrane is thought to be similar in nature to most other biological membranes and thus will only allow the escape of low-molecular-weight molecules into the cytoplasm.

Active targeting of polymer conjugates using receptor ligand targeting is also being investigated using targeting groups such as galactosamine. Currently a HPMA–doxorubicin–galactosamine conjugate (PK2) is in clinical trials. The galactose promotes the targeting of the asiaglycoprotein receptor selectively expressed on hepatocytes and hepatomas. Antibody targeting of conjugates is also a possibility (see section on antibody-targeted drug conjugates, above).

Polymer–drug conjugates

- *Xyotax.* In this polymer–drug conjugate, paclitaxel is conjugated to PGA via an ester linker. This conjugate has a high drug content (~37% w/w) and is stable in the circulation. The drug is released intracellularly via degradation of PGA by lysosomal proteases and the ester linker is degraded by esterases or acid hydrolysis. Xyotax is currently in clinical trials as a potential treatment for non-small-cell lung cancer and ovarian cancer.

Tip

Interferons are cytokines and interferon-alpha may be derived from leucocytes or lymphoblasts or through recombinant DNA technology. Subspecies of the human alpha gene are differentiated by a number, and further differentiated by a letter (e.g. interferon-alpha-2a) which indicates the amino acid sequences: interferon-alpha-2a has lysine at position 23 and histidine at 34, interferon alpha-2b has arginine at 23 and histidine at 34.

Polymer–protein conjugates

- *Oncaspar.* In this conjugate L-asparaginase is bound to non-biodegradable monomethoxyl PEG (5 kDa) via an amide linker. This conjugate is used for induction of remissions in acute lymphoblastic leukaemia. Asparaginase is an enzyme which breaks down the amino acid L-asparagine. This interferes with the growth of malignant cells which, unlike most healthy cells, are unable to synthesise L-asparagine for their metabolism. Following intravenous injection the plasma half-life of the native enzyme is 8–30 hours. Dosing regimens vary but generally require daily administration for 10 days. PEGylation of the protein increases its half-life to 5.7 days, markedly reducing the dosing regime. The PEGylated protein can also be used in patients who are hypersensitive to the native enzyme.

- *Neulasta.* This is a PEGylated granulocyte colony-stimulating factor. The monomethoxyl PEG has a molecular weight of 2 kDa and is bound to the active agent via an amide linker. This conjugate is available for the prevention of neutropenia associated with cancer and acquired immunodeficiency syndrome (AIDS) chemotherapy.
- *Pegasys.* In this conjugate interferon-alpha-2a is linked to a branched, non-biodegradable monomethyl PEG (40 kDa). It is also used as a monotherapy for chronic hepatitis B and for the treatment of chronic hepatitis C in combination with ribavirin (an antiviral nucleoside analogue) or as a monotherapy for chronic hepatitis C if ribavirin is not tolerated or is contraindicated.
- *Peg-Intron/ViraferonPeg.* This is a formulation of interferon-alpha-2b conjugated with monomethoxyl PEG via a carbamate linker. Cleavage of the active agent from the polymer occurs via β-lactamase or basic hydrolysis. The conjugate is given once weekly for 6–12 months as a monotherapy or in combination with ribavirin for the treatment of chronic hepatitis C.

Proteins as drug carriers

A variety of proteins, including glycoproteins, lysozyme and albumin, have also been investigated as potential carriers for drug targeting. However the main disadvantages of using these systems include their potential immunogenicity and physicochemical complexity, which complicate the preparation, purification and identification of the final conjugates formed. Proteins in general are difficult to formulate into a product as they can be degraded when exposed to a range of conditions including heat, freezing, light, pH extremes and shear stress. Yet formulations are available – dinileukin difitox (Ontak), a fusion protein of the cytokine interleukin-2 (IL-2) and the diphtheria toxin, is on the market. The cytokine moiety is responsible for the targeted transport of the toxin to IL-2 receptor overexpressing cells, such as cutaneous T-cell lymphomas. The binding

KeyPoint

- Proteins as drug carriers have also been investigated but their somewhat delicate structures and potential immunogenicity have limited their application.

of the protein to the receptor initiates the absorption into the cell where the diphtheria toxin causes cell death. A protein-based nanoparticulate delivery system has been approved and is discussed in the section on polymeric micelles as drug-targeting systems, below.

Polysaccharide carriers

Polysaccharides are generally also biodegradable and therefore avoid accumulation within the body. As with other soluble carriers, the physicochemical properties (molecular weight, electrical charge) of the polysaccharides are important factors dictating their pharmacokinetics. Of particular interest is the use of dextrans which are colloidal, hydrophilic molecules which are inert in biological media but in vivo are slowly hydrolysed to soluble sugars by dextranase.

KeyPoints

- Colloidal delivery systems can range from nanometres to several micrometres in size.
- These systems can generally carry more drug, and often do not need the drug to be conjugated to them.
- Drugs carried by these systems may be protected from degradation during transit to the target site.

Colloidal and particulate drug delivery systems

Particulate drug delivery systems can generally be described as constructs within the colloidal size range, which is roughly between 1 nm and 1 μm, and include dendrimers, nanoparticles, micelles, liposomes and microspheres. With these systems the drug is normally physically associated rather than covalently attached to the carrier, in contrast to the soluble carriers discussed above.

As mentioned in the section on soluble macromolecular drug carriers to promote targeting, above, the properties of a drug carrier can be changed by the conjugation of a drug. For example, if a significant change occurs to the overall size of the resulting conjugate this may limit the amount of drug carrier construct that can passively target specific sites. In addition, conjugates have a limited carrier capacity and therefore overall delivery is limited by both the capacity of the carrier to transport the drug and its access to the site. By contrast, particulate delivery systems offer the potential of higher drug loading, often without the need to modify the drug chemically or change the physical attributes of the carrier. Loading the drug within the delivery system can also offer enhanced protection against drug degradation. The high loading capacity of these systems therefore means that delivery of drug is less dictated by the volume of plasma extravasating to the target site. However their increased size compared to drug conjugates will influence their biodistribution.

Basic properties of colloidal and particulate delivery systems

The increased size of these systems compared to the conjugate delivery systems can offer advantages in increased drug loading and avoid chemical conjugation of the drug. However the particulate nature of these systems can result in rapid clearance from the systemic circulation due to the actions of the mononuclear phagocyte system (Chapter 7).

The size of these delivery systems can also limit their ability to leave the systemic circulation. In Chapter 7 it was discussed that a delivery system generally needs to leave the vasculature before it can reach its target. This requires the system to cross the endothelial lining of the blood circulation and for particulate drug delivery systems this is normally restricted to sites where the endothelial lining is fenestrated or sinusoidal and has a number of gaps between the cells, as in capillaries within the liver, spleen and bone marrow, or where the integrity of the endothelial barrier has been disturbed by inflammatory processes or by tumour growth.

Therefore we can see that the physicochemical properties of the particulate systems (including both their surface properties and size) will have a strong controlling effect on the pharmacokinetics and biodistribution of the delivery system.

KeyPoint

■ Particulates are cleared rapidly by cells of the MPS and the ability of larger particles to leave the systemic circulation is limited.

Designing particulate systems for passive targeting

Without modification of the surface properties, any delivery systems will be seen as 'foreign' by the immune system and will be opsonised and removed from the circulation by the MPS, leading to a rapid accumulation in the liver and spleen. This can be exploited if the target site is a part of the MPS such as the liver or spleen.

However to reach other target sites, clearance by the MPS must be avoided and therefore delivery systems should be formulated with sizes below 100 nm and with a hydrophilic polymer coating to avoid opsonisation. PEGylation of these systems by using PEG as a polymer coating is the most frequently adopted method to impart a hydrophilic coating on these systems. By increasing the surface hydrophilicity, PEGylation masks the surface characteristics

KeyPoints

■ To avoid MPS uptake particles need to be smaller than 100 nm and generally have a hydrophilic coat, leading to extended circulation times.
■ Avoiding MPS uptake can allow particles to accumulate in pathological sites with leaky vasculature.

Tip

As a guide, after intravenous injection most particulates, unless formulated to avoid MPS recognition, are rapidly cleared (in a matter of minutes) by macrophages of the MPS with maximal phagocytosis occurring with particles around 1–2 μm in diameter.

of the particulates (including charge or hydrophobicity), basically forming a shield over the surface of the particle which blocks interactions of opsonins with the particle surface. PEGylation of particles can be achieved by physical adsorption of a polymer on to a preformed particle or by chemically conjugating polymer chains on to the surface of the particle.

Therefore a hydrophilic coat combined with particle sizes below 100 nm allows for these delivery systems to:

- avoid the MPS
- have an extended blood circulation time
- accumulate in pathological sites with leaky vasculature due to their enhanced permeability and poor lymphatic drainage.

This applies to target sites, including tumours and sites of inflammation. Clinically most of the colloidal/particulate drug delivery systems available exploit passive targeting via the MPS or the EPR effect.

KeyPoint

- Active targeting requires avoiding MPS uptake, so the system has sufficient time within the circulation, and a targeting system.

Designing particulate systems for active targeting

To facilitate the active targeting of cell types, ligands specific to cell receptors/binding sites can be used. Examples of such targeting groups include antibodies, peptides, sugar groups and folate. These targeting groups can be conjugated directly on to the surface of the particulate system. However for active targeting a prolonged circulation time is also useful as it can provide more time for the delivery systems to reach and interact with the target. Therefore the targeting group can be conjugated to the end of the PEG polymer coating. This is sometimes referred to as functionalisation of the surface. There are many published studies demonstrating that the addition of targeting groups to long-circulating particulate delivery systems increases cell-specific targeting. However currently there are no active targeted particulate delivery systems available clinically.

KeyPoints

- Dendrimers are branched polymer macromolecules. As they are produced by controlled chemical synthesis they have a narrow size range.
- They can be designed for passive targeting with a PEG coat or for active targeting with the addition of targeting groups.
- Drugs can either be covalently bound to the dendrimer structure or solubilised within hydrophobic regions of the structure.

Dendrimers

Dendrimers are highly branched, monodisperse macromolecules. They have a regular and highly branched polymeric structure which can be between 1 and 100 nm in size, and thus they can be considered as macromolecules or nanoparticles. As they are built by controlled chemical synthesis we have included them within this section. Dendrimers can be seen as a further step in the evolution of polymeric systems from first linear structures through cross-linked and branched polymers but, unlike many polymers, dendrimers can be prepared to be nearly monodisperse in size with a large number of peripheral groups that may be used to bind the drug, PEG or a targeting group.

Dendrimers consist of three main architectural components: the core, the branches and the end groups (Figure 8.7) and can be prepared by a stepwise synthetic approach that adds branching multivalent monomer units to a core. The branching units are

Figure 8.7 Schematic representation of a dendrimer structure with encapsulated drug within the inner core or surface-bound. Targeting groups or solubilising groups such as poly(ethyleneglycol) can also be conjugated to the surface.

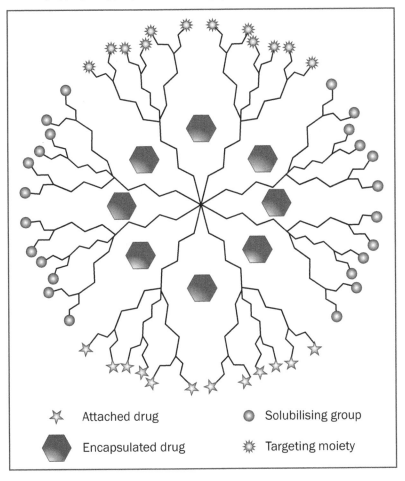

Attached drug   Solubilising group

Encapsulated drug   Targeting moiety

described as generations, starting with the central branched core molecule as generation 0 (G0) and increasing as each layer of branching is added (i.e. G1, G2). With the addition of each generation, the number of end groups available on the structure increases exponentially and the macromolecule tends to adopt a more globular shape with each generation (Figure 8.7).

As each of these components within the construct can be varied, this allows for dendrimers to be tailored in terms of their overall size, shape and functionality since all of these are determined by the chemical composition in terms of the core used, the interior branching and surface groups at the end of the molecular structure. Basically the molecular versatility of dendrimers is immense and they can be synthesised into a range of dimensions depending on the needs of the drug and the delivery site. Targeting groups can be added to the end of the dendrimer for active targeting or PEG groups can be added to modify the pharmacokinetics to promote passive targeting via the EPR effect. In general, the pharmacokinetics of these systems follow those already discussed with polymeric carriers and factors controlling their biodistribution include:

- Liver accumulation increases with dendrimer size.
- PEGylation significantly increases the half-life and decreases liver accumulation of these systems similar to other systems discussed.
- Dendrimers with <6 generations tend to accumulate in the kidney before excretion; larger dendrimers tend not to be filtered through this route.

Similar to polymeric carriers, dendrimers can be prepared to be biodegradable, and have a triggered drug release using linker groups, as discussed in the section on polymeric conjugates, above. However, as with polymeric systems in general, their drug-loading capacity can be limited. One benefit of using dendrimers as delivery systems is that they are single well-defined molecules, which gives advantages in terms of defining the products for manufacturing and quality control. This is an advantage over many self-assembly systems, such as micelles and liposomes, which are harder to define robustly as a product.

Currently dendrimers are being studied preclinically and the majority of studies have used dendrimers prepared from poly-amidoamine (PAMAM), poly-ethyleneimine and poly-L-lysine as building blocks. These systems have been shown to act as drug carriers where the drug can either be covalently bound to the dendrimer surface,

Tip

The polymer construct of the dendrimer will dictate if the system is biodegradable or not. Dendrimers prepared from amino acids, e.g. poly-L-lysine dendrimers, are biodegradable whereas PAMAM dendrimers are not degraded in vivo and are cleared via excretion.

or the drug can be solubilised within the hydrophobic core or pockets in the dendrimer structure. Similar to other targeted drug delivery systems, most efforts have been focused on enhancing the delivery of antineoplastic drugs and contrast agents. Studies have also investigated the use of dendrimers as drugs in their own right, with structures being designed with antiviral and antimicrobial properties.

Dendrimers are being investigated as possible delivery systems for a range of drugs, including anticancer agents such as doxorubin to improve their therapeutic profile. The conjugation of heavy metals such as gadolinium to dendrimers also offers the potential for these systems to be used as contrast agents and there has been a range of studies looking at their in vivo distribution after intravenous infusion.

Solid nanoparticles for drug delivery and targeting

In the widest sense a nanoparticle can be defined as a particle with one or more of its dimensions around 100 nm or less. By preparing these systems in the nanometre size range the properties of the nanoparticles are different from that of the bulk material. We have already discussed how the particle size of a delivery system will influence its pharmacokinetics and biodistribution. Therefore we can see that creating nanosized delivery systems can play an important role within drug delivery and targeting, particularly for chemotherapy agents through the EPR effect. There are a range of delivery systems that can be prepared to fit within the nanoscale range, including polymeric systems, dendrimers, micelles, liposomes and nanoparticles prepared from a range of substances. We have already discussed polymer conjugate systems and dendrimers so within this section we will mainly focus on solid nanoparticles. Solid nanoparticles can be constructed in a variety of ways, including nanosizing of solid drug particles, and the formulation of polymeric nanoparticles, protein nanoparticles and solid lipid nanoparticles. Like the other delivery systems already discussed, nanoparticle systems can be used to address the three main issues

KeyPoints

- Nanotechnology generally refers to systems of around 100 nm in size or less.
- There are a range of drug delivery systems that fit within this definition, including macromolecules and colloidal/particulate systems.

Tip

The establishment of the term nanotechnology has resulted from the development of new systems (e.g. nanotubes) and also from the rebranding of older colloidal systems (e.g. micelles and liposomes). In the most basic sense, nanotechnology can incorporate any delivery system in the nanometre range which can include micelles, polymer particulates and liposomes. However some of these systems can also be prepared as larger carrier systems. So, for example, in some instances a liposome system may be considered as nanotechnology and in other instances as a larger particulate system depending on the size of liposomes made.

Tip

Solid drug nanoparticles can be made directly as dry powder systems but they have limited physical stability due to their high surface free energy and generally rapidly aggregate on storage. To avoid this, nanoparticles need to be formulated with additional excipients to reduce their agglomeration (see Chapter 2 for further details).

KeyPoints

- Polymeric nanoparticles can be formulated to take advantage of the EPR effect.
- To prepare polymeric nanoparticles poly(lactide-co-glycolide) (PLGA), polylactic acid (PLA) and polycaprolactone (PCL) are commonly used polymers.

hindering drug development: low solubility, poor bioavailability and/or toxicity. The use of nanoparticles to improve solubility and dissolution rate has been discussed in Chapter 2 and within this section we will focus on their ability to improve the efficacy and safety of drugs through enhanced delivery and targeting.

Solid polymeric nanoparticles

Solid polymeric nanoparticles are prepared using a wide variety of either natural or synthetic polymers. The most commonly studied are biodegradable polymers such as PLGA, PLA, PCL and polysaccharides (particularly chitosan). These polymers are well characterised and in particular PLGA is used in a range of clinical products. Following introduction into the body, copolymers of polylactic and glycolic acid undergo hydrolysis, forming the biologically compatible and metabolisable moieties lactic acid and glycolic acid, which are eventually removed from the body by the citric acid cycle. In terms of drug delivery the main areas in which these systems are being investigated is for passive targeting of drugs to tumour sites via the EPR effect. To produce 'stealth' nanoparticles, PEG PLGA copolymers are often employed to extend the circulation time. Active targeting of these systems by the attachment of targeting groups to the nanoparticles has also been investigated.

PLGA has been widely tested for toxicity and safety and is currently used in humans for resorbable sutures and implants. Eligard, although not an example of a targeted system, is an example of a PLGA polymeric matrix suspension formulated to give controlled release of leuprolide acetate over a 1-, 3-, 4- or 6-month period. After subcutaneous injection it forms a solid drug delivery depot.

Polymeric nanoparticles can be prepared by a solvent evaporation method where the polymer and drug to be loaded within the nanoparticles are dissolved in a solvent such as dichloromethane. The solvent is then emulsified to produce globules in the nanometre size range and the solvent is subsequently evaporated off to produce nanoparticles as a suspension. A multiple emulsion (water-in-oil-in-water: w/o/w) method can also be used where the drug in an aqueous phase is emulsified within a solvent polymer phase. This first emulsion is then added to a second aqueous phase to produce the double emulsion. The solvent is then evaporated off under reduced pressure to produce nanoparticles. In both methods the particle size will be dependent on the emulsification process but the latter method can be beneficial if the drug is liable to degradation/denaturation when in contact with a solvent, e.g. in the case of proteins. However, in both methods proteins may be damaged during the emulsification stages. Also for large-scale production of polymeric particles, solvent evaporation is not ideal as ensuring removal of the solvent to safe levels may be difficult. For both types of preparation drug entrapment and release profile from these nanoparticles will be influenced by the drug incorporated and the polymer used.

Solid protein nanoparticles

Proteins can also be used for the construction of nanoparticles, and the first commercial product based on protein nanotechnology is Abraxane (nab-paclitaxel). Abraxane consists of 130 nm particles of albumin-bound paclitaxel. It is supplied as a lyophilised powder for reconstitution into an injectable suspension using 0.9% sodium chloride. Abraxane was approved by the US Food and Drug Administration in January 2005 for the treatment of breast cancer in patients who do not respond to combination chemotherapy for metastatic disease or relapse within 6 months of adjuvant chemotherapy. Abraxane is the first Cremophor-free paclitaxel product. By avoiding the use of Cremophor, this formulation potentially offers to overcome the toxicity problems associated with the use of Cremophor.

> ## KeyPoints
>
> - Nanoparticles can be prepared from proteins and there is an albumin-based system clinically available.
> - The albumin in the formulation acts to stabilise the system and may promote passage across the endothelial lining and tumour targeting.

However the albumin within the nanoparticle albumin technology (nab) used in Abraxane has several roles, some of which are particularly appropriate for targeted drug delivery in oncology. From a physicochemical point of view, albumin functions to coat the paclitaxel and provide colloidal stabilisation to the drug. Albumin is able to do so due to its ability reversibly and non-covalently to bind hydrophobic substances. In addition to this, albumin may play a role in supporting active targeting of the drug to tumour cells. Within the body, albumin is able to transport hydrophobic molecules such as vitamins, hormones and other plasma constituents and deliver these substances across the endothelial lining and out of the blood into the extravascular space via endothelial transcytosis. This process is receptor-mediated, with albumin binding to gp60 glycoprotein receptors on the cell surface. This prompts the binding of the internal protein, caveolin-1, to the inner side of the cell membrane which subsequently results in the internalisation of the cell membrane and the formation of a transcytotic vesicle. These vesicles, referred to as caveolae, transport their contents (in this case the albumin-bound paclitaxel) across the endothelial cell lining into the extravascular space.

This albumin gp60-mediated uptake may also play a role in preferential intratumour accumulation of paclitaxel, which was found to be 33% higher for nab-paclitaxel compared with a Cremophor-based formulation. Tumour cells may show an up-regulation of gp60 and, once the nanoparticles are in the interstitium, the albumin may bind to an extracellular matrix glycoprotein known as SPARC (secreted protein acid and rich in cysteine), which is also overexpressed in tumour cells. This may result in the delivery of paclitaxel directly to the tumour cell. Given that this mechanism is an attribute of the albumin carrier system and not the drug, it is conceivable it may be applied to the delivery of other low-solubility anticancer agents.

Paclitaxel and Cremophor EL

Several anticancer agents are hydrophobic in nature (e.g. paclitaxel) and rely on drug delivery systems to improve their solubility. Indeed, the clinical development of paclitaxel was originally delayed because of problems in drug formulation. Solvent-based delivery systems for intravenous administration of such drugs are generally used for the treatment in many solid tumours. Paclitaxel is available as Taxol, a liquid formulation where paclitaxel is dissolved in polyethoxylated caster oil (Cremophor EL) and ethanol. However this formulation requires special infusion sets, prolonged infusion times (3 hours) and premedication with corticosteroids and antihistamines to reduce the risk of hypersensitivity reactions. Cremophor EL has also been associated with neutropenia and peripheral neuropathy. Besides the toxicity issues, these delivery systems may reduce tumour penetration of the drug through the formation of large polar micelles.

Solid lipid nanoparticles

Solid lipid nanoparticles are colloidal particles made of solid lipids (e.g. solid triglycerides, saturated phospholipids and fatty acids) dispersed in an aqueous phase. In contrast to oil-in-water emulsions, in which the dispersed oil phase is liquid, this avoids the potential for droplet coalescence and may provide a better protection of the drug incorporated into the lipid particles against chemical and enzymatic degradation, as well as prolonged drug release. Usually the size of the

KeyPoints

- Solid lipid nanoparticles are composed of high-melting-point lipids.
- As with other nanoparticles, stealth coating offers the potential to target these systems passively.

dispersed lipid particles is in the range of 50 to several hundreds of nanometres, making them suitable for intravenous applications.

Typically solid lipid nanoparticles are produced by either hot or cold homogenisation. In hot homogenisation, the lipid matrix is molten and the lipophilic drug is dissolved in the molten lipids. This lipid phase is then dispersed into a hot-water phase which usually contains surfactants as stabilisers for the lipid particles. The warm dispersion is then homogenised at high pressure to produce initially a nanoemulsion which is then cooled down to allow the recrystallisation of the lipid phase, resulting in formation of a solid lipid nanoparticle dispersion. Cold homogenisation is used to produce solid lipid nanoparticles containing hydrophilic drugs. Here the drug is dispersed in the molten lipid phase which is then allowed to cool down. The solid matrix is then dispersed by a high-pressure homogenisation process into the aqueous phase. It is also possible to prepare solid lipid nanoparticle dispersions by dissolving the lipids in ethanol and injecting them into a warm aqueous phase followed by ultrasonication to reduce particle size and cooling to solidify the lipid phase.

Solid lipid nanoparticle dispersions have been developed for parenteral, oral, ocular, dermal and cosmetic applications, but recently have also been investigated as a potential delivery system for targeted drug delivery. PEG coating of these systems has been shown to target tumour sites passively via the EPR effect. To target cancer cells actively, covalently coupling ferritin to the lipids used in the formulation of the solid lipid nanoparticles has been tested. Galactose has also been investigated to target liver carcinoma cells, which have increased levels of galactose receptor molecules. However the development of solid lipid nanoparticles for targeted delivery is still at a very early stage (in vitro and animal experiments) and no products have reached the market. It is also to date not clear if this approach has a significant advantage over other colloidal delivery systems.

Inorganic nanoparticles

There is a range of nanoparticles that have been fabricated from inorganic materials including carbon nanotubes, ceramics, metals, metal oxides and metal sulfides. Calcium phosphate-based nanoshells have also been prepared which have a hollow reservoir which can be loaded with drug. The inorganic systems are generally stable and can be used to entrap and protect drugs; however generally they are not biodegradable so their application as potential pharmaceutical products is limited.

Polymeric micelles as drug-targeting systems

A wide range of molecules with surfactant properties are known to self-assemble in an aqueous environment to form micelle structures.

KeyPoints

- Micelles can be used to deliver poorly soluble drugs and can be formulated from surfactants and block copolymers.
- Polymeric micelles are generally more stable than surfactant micelles and can have a hydrophilic coat to promote 'stealth' properties.
- Targeting groups can also be conjugated to the surface of the micelles.

The driving force for micelle formation is through a combination of intermolecular forces, including hydrophobic, electrostatic and hydrogen bonding. Their small size and colloidal stability mean that they are not subject to particle aggregation.

A mixed micellar formulation of amphotericin B deoxycholate (Fungazone) is available for parenteral administration. Amphotericin B is a potent antifungal agent used to treat invasive fungal infections such as systemic candidiasis and histoplasmosis, but amphotericin B has very low oral bioavailability. However, parenteral administration is associated with severe side-effects, including haemolysis and nephrotoxicity. In addition to Fungazone there are three formulations available for amphotericin B: a liposome system, a lipid-based system and a formulation where the drug is formulated in a complex with cholesteryl sulfate. Whilst the liposome and lipid complex systems can reduce toxicity by modifying the pharmacokinetic and pharmacodynamic properties of the drug, the mixed micellar formulation does not improve tolerability of amphotericin B and does not offer any control over the delivery of the drug.

For the delivery and targeting of drugs, block copolymers with amphiphilic properties (due to large solubility differences between their hydrophilic and hydrophobic groups) have been widely investigated. Compared to surfactant micelles, polymeric micelles are generally more stable and have low critical micellar concentrations. With these polymeric systems a variety of hydrophilic components – in particular, PEG – is used for the outer shell of the micelle. These hydrophilic polymer blocks not only provide the hydrophilic component of the molecule supporting the formation of micelles but they also provide steric stabilisation and stealth coating to the constructs. The hydrophobic component of these polymeric micelles can comprise polyaspartate, polylactide or polycaprolactone. Polymeric micelles generally have sizes from 5 nm up to as large as 100 nm and have a narrow particle size distribution. They are therefore sometimes referred to as nanoparticles. In terms of drug delivery, various types of drugs can be incorporated within the inner core of the micelles, by either chemical conjugation or physical entrapment (Figure 8.8).

Due to these attributes, polymeric micelles can be used as drug-targeting systems as they can offer a high drug-loading capacity and are able to control the biodistribution of the drug through the tailoring of their size and surface characteristics. Due to their

Figure 8.8 Block copolymer used to prepare a micelle and the resultant micelle.

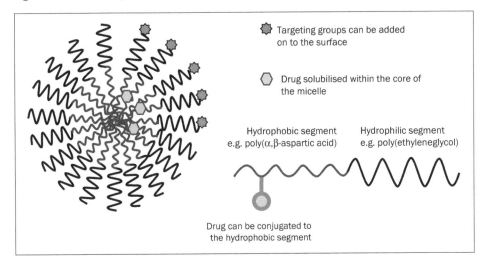

Targeting groups can be added on to the surface

Drug solubilised within the core of the micelle

Hydrophobic segment
e.g. poly(α,β-aspartic acid)

Hydrophilic segment
e.g. poly(ethyleneglycol)

Drug can be conjugated to the hydrophobic segment

particle size, after intravenous injection, micelles are unable to pass through the epithelia of normal vessels but they are able to target tumour sites passively due to the EPR effect. Clinical trials investigating the application of polymeric micelles to target paclitaxel, cisplatin and camptothecin passively via the EPR effect are currently under way.

Actively targeted micellar systems have also been investigated. The addition of targeting moieties such as folate, sugar residues or proteins to the end of the block copolymers has been shown in animal studies to promote receptor-mediated targeting of the micelle systems. For example, the chemical attachment of monoclonal antibodies to reactive groups incorporated in the hydrophilic coating of polymeric micelles can promote specific interactions of the micelles with corresponding antigens. These micelles are often referred to as immunomicelles but currently these systems are still limited to preclinical research.

Examples of polymeric micellar systems

- *Genexol-PM.* This is a polymeric micelle formulation of paclitaxel prepared using methoxy-PEG-poly(D,L-lactide). In vivo antitumour efficacy of the micellar formulation was significantly higher than that of Taxol. Genexol-PM obtained a premarket approval in Korea in July 2006 and clinical trials are ongoing.
- *Paclitaxel-incorporating micelles (NK105).* NK105 micelles contain block copolymers built from polyethylene glycol and polyaspartate. The molecular weight of the polymer is 20 kDa in total, with a PEG component of 12 kDa. The paclitaxel is physically entrapped within the core of the micelle through

hydrophobic interactions with the polyaspartate and the formulation contains ~23% w/w of the drug. In mouse studies NK105 exhibited slower clearance from the plasma than free drug with the half-life in plasma being approximately 5 times longer when the drug was delivered using the polymer micelle formulation and concentrations at the tumour site were increased two- to threefold with the polymeric micelles.

■ *Cisplatin-incorporating micelles (NC-6004)*. Similar to paclitaxel, cisplatin is an anticancer agent with a major side-effect profile which includes nephrotoxicity and neurotoxicity. NC-6004 is prepared from PEG-poly(sodium-L-glutamate) block copolymer. The PEG forms the outer hydrophilic shell. The hydrophobic core of the micelle contains cisplatin complexed with the PGA component of the copolymer. The overall weight of the copolymer is 18 kDa with a 12 kDa PEG contribution. These micelles are 30 nm in size and have a very low critical micelle concentration and thus have a high stability. The interactions between the drug and the polymer within the micelle core have been attributed to the stability of these systems. Similar to the NK105 micelles, these micelles improved circulation time and enhanced tumour targeting of the drug, thereby reducing the side-effect profile.

KeyPoint

■ Microemulsions can be formulated to solubilise and target anticancer agents to tumour sites via the EPR effect.

Microemulsions for drug targeting

Oil-in-water microemulsions are a useful delivery system for the parenteral delivery of hydrophobic drugs. As discussed in Chapter 2, their ability to form spontaneously, ease of manufacture and high solubilisation capacity make them ideal vehicles. The globule size of microemulsions is less than 150 nm so generally they could be seen to fit within the loose description of nanotechonology and the small size of the microemulsion can result in longer circulation times, particularly when suitable excipients such as PEGylated surfactants are employed to provide a 'stealth' surface coating. As with other 'stealth' nanodelivery systems, passive targeting can be achieved: in preclinical trials PEGylated phospholipid-based microemulsions were able to provide long circulation times, enhanced concentrations of vincristine (a hydrophobic cytotoxic alkaloid) in the tumour and reduced concentrations of vincristine in the heart, spleen and liver compared to 'free' vincristine.

Liposomes and surfactant-based vesicles

Liposomes are closed spherical vesicles consisting of an aqueous core surrounded by one or more concentrically arranged bilayer membranes (Figure 8.9). These membranes can be composed of natural or synthetic lipid molecules. Usually phospholipids are employed to formulate liposomes; however a range of other polar lipids can be used to form bilayer constructs. Liposomes were the first of the parenteral particulate drug delivery systems to be approved for clinical use and a number of liposome products are available for clinical use. Like the other particulate delivery systems already discussed, liposomes can protect the entrapped drug from degradation and change the biodistribution of the drug by promoting passive targeting of the drug or active targeting through the addition of targeting groups to the liposome surface.

KeyPoints

- Liposomes are bilayer vesicles generally composed of phospholipids.
- They can entrap hydrophilic drugs within their aqueous core and lipophilic drugs within the lipid bilayers.
- They can be prepared in a range of sizes with single or multiple bilayers.
- There are several liposome formulations used in clinical practice.

Additional advantages of using liposomes as drug delivery systems include their ability to encapsulate both hydrophilic drugs within the aqueous regions of the system (e.g. Myocet) and solubilise lipophilic drugs within their bilayer regions (e.g. AmBisome). Through modification of the bilayer composition, the drug release rate of entrapped drugs can also be controlled. Examples of liposomal systems currently available are given in Table 8.3.

Liposomes have been investigated as delivery systems for a wide range of routes from ocular to anal, with some being more realistic than others. As can be seen in Table 8.3, the main application of

Figure 8.9 Schematic representation of a lipid which can form bilayer vesicles with drug entrapped in the aqueous phase or the bilayer. PEG, poly(ethyleneglycol).

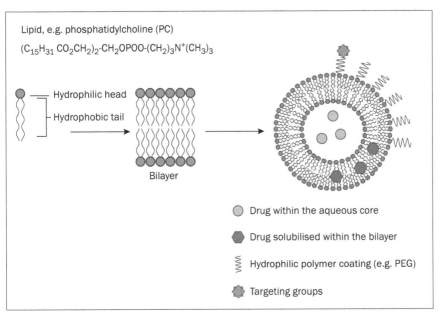

Lipid, e.g. phosphatidylcholine (PC)

$(C_{15}H_{31} CO_2CH_2)_2\text{-}CH_2OPOO\text{-}(CH_2)_3N^+(CH_3)_3$

Hydrophilic head
Hydrophobic tail

Bilayer

Drug within the aqueous core

Drug solubilised within the bilayer

Hydrophilic polymer coating (e.g. PEG)

Targeting groups

Table 8.3 Examples of liposome products currently available

Trade name	Drug	Description	Indications
Caelyx/ Doxil	Doxorubicin	80–100 nm sterically stabilised liposomes composed of pegylated distearoyl phosphatidyl ethanolamine, hydrogenated soy phosphatidylcholine and cholesterol	Advanced ovarian cancerAdvanced breast cancerAIDS-related Kaposi's sarcoma
DaunoXome	Daunorubicin	~45 nm-sized liposomes composed of distearoyl phosphatidylcholine and cholesterol	Kaposi's sarcoma
Myocet	Doxorubicin	150–190 nm-sized liposomes composed of egg phosphatidylcholine and cholesterol	First-line treatment of metastatic breast cancer in women
Depocyt	Cytarabine	These are multivesicle liposomes composed of dioleoylphosphatidylcholine (DOPC), cholesterol, triolein, and dipalmitoylphosphatidylglycerol (DPPG). The vesicles range in size from 3 to 30 μm	Intrathecal treatment of lymphomatous meningitis
AmBisome	Amphotericin B	These vesicles are < 100 nm in size, and are composed of soy phosphatidylcholine, cholesterol, distearoylphosphatidylglycerol	Systemic fungal infections
Epaxal	Formalin inactivated hepatitis A virus	These are 150 nm virosomes composed of purified influenza virus surface antigens phosphatidycholine and phosphatidylethanolamine	Hepatitis A vaccine
Inflexal V Berna	Purified influenza haemagglutinin glycoprotein and neuraminidase	Virosome system similar to epaxal	Influenza vaccine
Visudyne	Verteporfin	Dimyristoyl phosphatidylcholine (DMPC) and egg phosphatidylglycerol (PG)	Photodynamic therapy for macular degradation

Many of these systems are discussed in more detail in the text.
AIDS, acquired immunodeficiency syndrome.

Tip

There are a range of vesicle-based formulations and lipid complexes available. Not all of these may be defined as liposomes in a stricter sense, e.g. some lipid complex systems do not have an aqueous core but are sometimes referred to as liposome-based systems.

liposomes has been to enhance delivery and targeting of drugs with harsh side-effect profiles. The second main area of application has been as vaccine adjuvants. Therefore the examples and case studies discussed below will focus on these two clinical roles.

Lipid formulations of amphotericin B

Amphotericin B has a broad spectrum of activity and is generally the drug of choice for life-threatening invasive fungal infections, including disseminated candidiasis, aspergillosis and protozoal infections affecting the internal organs (visceral leishmaniasis). However, its use is compromised by associated adverse side-effects.

Lipid formulations of the drug offer a better therapeutic index and there are three commercially available lipid formulations of amphotericin B in clinical use: AmBisome, Abelcet and Amphotec.

- *AmBisome.* This is a small unilamellar liposome formulation with a well-defined size range of ~80 nm. Due to its aqueous core this can be described as the only 'true' liposome formulation of the three products. It is composed of hydrogenated soy phosphatidylcholine, cholesterol, distearoylphosphatidylglycerol and amphotericin B in a 2:1:0.8:0.4 molar ratio. It also contains α-tocopherol as an antioxidant. The drug is intercalated within the liposomal membrane.
- *Abelcet.* This formulation is composed of amphotericin B, dimyristoyl phosphatidylcholine and dimyristoyl phosphatidylglycerol in a 1:1 drug-to-lipid molar ratio. It forms ribbon-like complexes which due to their structure are difficult to size but have been reported to be around 1.6–11 μm in diameter, with 90% of the particles being smaller than 6 μm.
- *Amphotec.* This formulation consists of amphotericin B in a complex with cholesteryl sulfate at a 1:1 molar ratio to form stable colloidal disc-like structures with diameters of 100–140 nm in size.

All these formulations contain amphotericin B and all three lipid formulations offer a better therapeutic index by reducing amphotericin toxicity. The three formulations, however, differ in shape and size and subsequently in their pharmacokinetic profile (including clearance, volume of distribution, C_{max} and area under the concentration curve). In terms of clinical safety, when used at similar doses (5 mg/kg), Abelcet caused significantly higher rates of side-effects (including chills/rigors, fevers, hypoxia and other infusion-related reactions) than AmBisome. Nephrotoxicity was also significantly higher with Abelcet compared to AmBisome. Comparison of the clinical efficacy of the various systems seems to suggest that the lipid-based formulations are superior to the non-lipid formulation, but since the tolerated dose of these formulations varies, further studies, including those on cost-effectiveness, are needed.

Liposome formation

In aqueous systems lipid molecules can self-assemble into various structures, including micelles, inverted micelles, liquid crystals (hexagonal phases, lamellar phases, cubic phases) as well as dispersed liquid crystalline structures, of which liposomes (dispersed lamellar structures) are the most important. The fact that liposomes may be regarded as dispersed lamellar phases also means that to prepare liposomes energy has to be added into the systems to allow for their dispersion.

KeyPoint

- The geometrical shape of polar lipid molecules dictates how they self-aggregate and determines the resulting structure of the aggregate.

The driving forces for self-assembly of the lipids are to allow the hydrophilic regions of the lipids to interact with the aqueous phase and the hydrophobic regions of the molecules to be segregated away from the hydrophilic phase. The formation of these structures is dependent on the temperature, lipid concentration and electrostatic interactions of the polar lipids with the solvent and solute molcules. However the type of aggregate a specific amphiphile forms is to a large extent dictated by its molecular shape, as this will influence its geometrical packing properties in a given solution environment. The shape of the lipid may be expressed as its critical packing parameter (p), which can be defined as:

$$p = \frac{v}{a_o l_c}$$

where:

- p is the critical packing parameter
- v is the molecular volume of the hydrophobic part of the polar lipid
- a_o is the surface area per molecule at the hydrocarbon–water interface
- l_c is the length of the hydrocarbon region.

For polar lipids with $p < 1/3$, spherical micelles are formed. For p values between 1/3 and 1/2, cylindrical micelles are formed. As the hydrophobic tail region of the lipid increases in volume (e.g. with double-chained lipids), flexible bilayer vesicles form. A further increase in the ratio of head group area to tail region promotes the formation of planar bilayers or inverted micelles (Figure 8.10). This is a simple but useful approach to predicting the self-assembling structures lipids tend to form. However changes in pH, temperature and lipid concentration can affect these states of aggregation and, furthermore, aggregates can interact to form larger structures. Also, mixtures of lipids can allow for liposomes to be formed from lipids that do not have the desired truncated cone shape. By using combinations of differently shaped lipids, a bilayer structure can be stabilised and liposomes can be formulated. However, in all cases, liposomes do not disperse spontaneously and energy must be added to the system to drive the formation of the liposome constructs.

Commonly employed lipids in liposome products

There are a large number of lipids used to prepare liposomes, but most commonly phospholipids are employed, in particular phosphatidylcholines. Phosphatidylcholines, also referred to as lecithin, can be derived from both natural and synthetic sources. Commonly they are extracted from egg yolk and soya bean. They are the principal phospholipid used in liposome formulations because of their low cost relative to other lipids and because of their neutral (zwitter-ionic) charge and chemical inertness.

Figure 8.10 The critical packing parameter of example lipids and the structures they form.

Lipid	Critical packing parameter	Shape	Structure formed
Single-chain lipids with large head group areas e.g. Sodium dodecylsulphate	$< \frac{1}{3}$	Cone 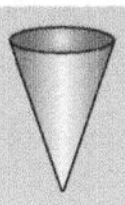	Spherical micelles 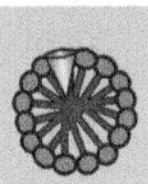
Single-chain lipids with small head group areas e.g. Cetyltrimethylammonium bromide	$\frac{1}{3}$ to $\frac{1}{2}$	Truncated cone 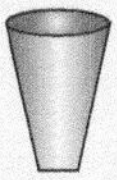	Cylindrical micelles 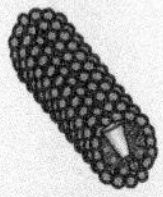
Double-chain lipids with large head groups e.g. Phosphatidylcholine	$\frac{1}{2}$ to 1	Truncated cone 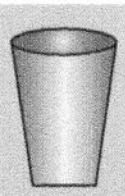	Bilayer vesicles 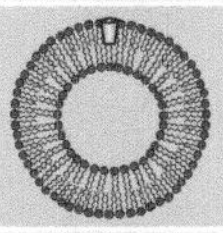
Double-chain lipids with small head groups e.g. Phosphatidyl-ethanolamine	~1	Cylinder 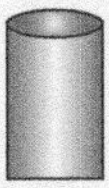	Planar bilayers 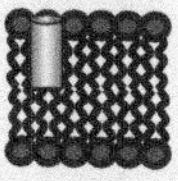
Double-chain lipids with small head groups and unsaturated chain tails e.g. Dioleoyl phosphatidyl-ethanolamine	>1	Inverted truncated cone 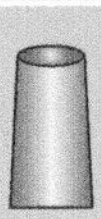	Inverted micelles 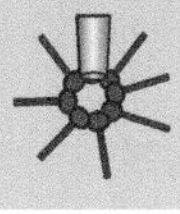

Phospholipids can have a range of head and tail groups (Figure 8.11). The choice of head group will influence the surface charge of the liposomes; commonly employed phospholipids include:

■ phosphatidylcholine and phosphatidylethanolamine, which are zwitter-ionic in nature
■ phosphatidylglycerol and phosphatidylserine, which have a negatively charged head group.

The tail of the phospholipid is also important for the characteristics of the liposome systems. The carbon chain length and the degree of saturation influence the transition temperature of the lipid: dimyristoylphosphatidylcholine has a transition temperature of 23 °C compared to distearoylphosphatidylcholine, which has a much higher transition temperature (55 °C).

Cholesterol is a major component of natural membranes and is also commonly used in liposomal products. Its incorporation into liposome bilayers significantly affects the liposome properties. Cholesterol does not form bilayers on its own but can be

KeyPoints

■ Phosphatidylcholine is a commonly used component in liposomes; however a range of other lipids are also used.
■ The lipid head group dictates the surface charge of the liposomes.
■ The lipid acyl tail influences the melting point of the lipid bilayer and its permeability and therefore influences drug release rates from liposomes.
■ The presence of cholesterol within the bilayers can reduce their permeability and drug leakage.

Figure 8.11 Examples of phospholipid structures.

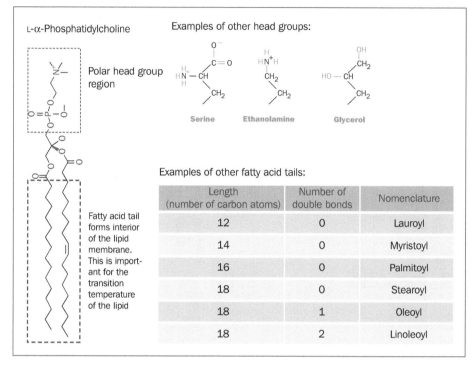

L-α-Phosphatidylcholine   Examples of other head groups:

Polar head group region

Serine   Ethanolamine   Glycerol

Fatty acid tail forms interior of the lipid membrane. This is important for the transition temperature of the lipid

Examples of other fatty acid tails:

Length (number of carbon atoms)	Number of double bonds	Nomenclature
12	0	Lauroyl
14	0	Myristoyl
16	0	Palmitoyl
18	0	Stearoyl
18	1	Oleoyl
18	2	Linoleoyl

Tip

Lethicin from natural sources is a mixture of phosphatidylcholines, with chains of different lengths and varying degrees of unsaturation.

incorporated into phospholipid membranes at concentrations up to 50%. Being amphipathic in nature, cholesterol inserts itself into the membrane with its hydroxyl group oriented towards the aqueous layers and the rigid steroid tail next to the carbons of the phospholipid chains. The presence of cholesterol in the bilayer influences the freedom of movement of the phospholipid acyl chains and at higher concentrations can reduce the bilayer permeability of the liposomes, thereby improving drug retention. The presence of cholesterol within liposome formulations has also been shown to improve stability of liposomes in vivo. This may be a result of the cholesterol limiting the freedom of movements of the phospholipids in the bilayer, and reducing the loss of these lipids to lipoproteins. This loss of lipids results in permeable bilayers, which lead to drug leakage and opsonisation and therefore should be avoided.

Alternatives to lipid-based vesicles

In addition to phospholipid-based vesicles, a range of alternative surfactants have also been incorporated into bilayer constructs, leading to a range of related systems, including the following.

- *Non-ionic surfactant vesicles or niosomes.* These vesicles are prepared using non-ionic surfactants rather than phospholipids so may offer advantages in terms of chemical stability. Like liposomes, they can be prepared in a range of sizes and incorporate drugs in a similar fashion to liposomes. Currently these systems are used in cosmetic products.
- *Bilosomes.* Bilosomes are an extension of the non-ionic surfactant vesicles where bile salts such as deoxycholate are added to the formulation. The presence of these bile salts enhances the stability for delivery via the oral route by protecting them from disruption by digestive enzymes in the gastric environment. These systems are being investigated for oral delivery of a range of drugs, in particular as systems to support the oral delivery of subunit vaccines, since they can be taken up by the gut lymphatics to produce both systemic and mucosal immune responses.
- *Polymerised liposomes.* Polymerisation of the liposome bilayer can also enhance the stability of liposomes via the oral route and research has investigated their potential for delivery of peptides, proteins and vaccines orally.
- *Virosomes.* These are liposomes prepared from influenza virus and envelope material rather than phospholipids; they contain functional viral envelope proteins. They are small unilamellar vesicles (150 nm) composed of influenza virus haemagglutinin, neuraminidase, phosphatidylcholine and phosphatidylethanolamine. Due to their bilayer composition they can be used as effective vaccines. Virosome-based vaccines are available on the market (see section on liposomes as vaccine delivery systems).
- *Lipoplexes.* A range of cationic lipids have been investigated for their ability to promote the delivery of genetic material to support gene therapy strategies. Within these systems cationic small unilamellar

Tips

The transition temperature of lipids is defined as the temperature above which the lipid physical state changes from the ordered gel phase (where the hydrocarbon tails of the lipid are fully extended and closely packed) to the disordered liquid crystalline phase (where the hydrocarbon chains are randomly oriented). This liquid crystalline phase is fluid and generally results in the bilayer being more permeable. Factors which affect the phase transition temperature include:
- Hydrocarbon chain length: as length increases, phase transition temperature increases, as longer chains have high van der Waals interactions and more energy is required to disrupt them.
- Degree of saturation: introducing a double bond into the tail reduces van der Waals interactions so less energy is required to disrupt them.

KeyPoints

- Vesicles can be prepared from a range of lipids, not just phospholipids.
- Examples include vesicles prepared from non-ionic surfactants, bile salts, viral membrane components, cationic surfactants and polymerised lipids.

vesicles are formed and complexed with anionic DNA. This results in the electrostatic binding of the DNA to the cationic liposomes to form lipoplexes which can enhance the delivery of plasmid DNA. These systems are highly efficient in vitro yet generally suffer from low efficacy in vivo.

Overall these systems are prepared in similar ways to liposomes and generally display many similar traits to liposomal systems.

KeyPoints

- Liposomes can be classified based on their composition or based on their size and number of bilayers.
- MLV are large multilamellar vesicles.
- SUV are small unilamellar vesicles.
- LUV are large unilamellar vesicles.

Classification and nomenclature of liposomes

There are various ways of classifying liposomes, including classification based on their composition and in vivo application:

- 'Stealth' liposomes, which have a PEG coat
- Immunoliposomes, which have an antibody-targeting moiety
- Cationic liposomes prepared using positively charged lipids.

However the most widely accepted nomenclature for lipid vesicles is that originally agreed upon at the 1978 New York Academy of Sciences meeting. This is to classify liposomes into three main types, based on their size and number of bilayers (Figure 8.12), as follows.

- *Multilamellar vesicles.* These are vesicles which consist of a large number of concentric bilayers. Their size ranges from 100 nm to several micrometres, depending on their composition and their

Figure 8.12 Liposome types.

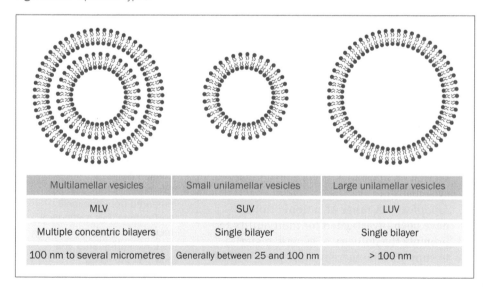

Multilamellar vesicles	Small unilamellar vesicles	Large unilamellar vesicles
MLV	SUV	LUV
Multiple concentric bilayers	Single bilayer	Single bilayer
100 nm to several micrometres	Generally between 25 and 100 nm	> 100 nm

method of preparation. They are easy to make in the laboratory; however their larger size (and generally wide size distribution) limits their application in vivo. Due to their multiple bilayers they have a relatively low encapsulation capacity for hydrophilic molecules and are better suited to encapsulation of lipophilic substances.

■ *Small unilamellar vesicles.* These vesicles consist of a single bilayer enclosing an aqueous core and theoretically can be as small as ~25 nm. However, more commonly this term is used to describe vesicles between 25 and 100 nm. They are generally more homogeneous in size than multilamellar vesicles, making them useful for parenteral drug delivery. Due to their small size they have a large surface curvature and a high membrane tension. Their small size does result in a low ratio of internal aqueous volume per mole of lipid.

■ *Large unilamellar vesicles.* These are single bilayer liposomes, generally over 100 nm in size. Due to their size, they have a larger aqueous core than small unilamellar vesicles so in comparison can entrap high amounts of hydrophilic drugs.

Preparation of liposomes

There are a range of methods employed for the preparation of liposomes. The choice of method to use will depend on the scale of manufacture, the lipids employed in the formulation, the drug to be incorporated and the size of liposomes required. However in a very general sense liposomes are formed from the hydration of dry lipids, and these liposomes can be reduced in size by the addition of energy to disrupt the bilayer structures to form smaller vesicles. This can be achieved via homogenisation, sonication or extrusion. An example of a convenient small-scale method for the preparation of liposomes (commonly referred to as the 'lipid hydration' method or 'hand-shaken' method) can be summarised as follows:

■ Bilayer-forming compounds are mixed in a volatile organic solvent mixture (e.g. chloroform:methanol, 9:1 v/v).

■ Drugs to be incorporated within the bilayer should also be added to the solvent mixture.

■ The solvent is removed by rotary evaporation under reduced pressure to prepare a dry lipid film.

■ An appropriate volume of aqueous buffer is added to the dry film (containing any hydrophilic drug to be incorporated). This should be done at temperatures above the transition temperature of the main lipid component within the liposome formulation.

■ Finally agitation of the film to force the lipids into liposome structures will promote formation of multilamellar vesicles. These liposomes can then be reduced in size via a range of methods such as sonication or extrusion.

KeyPoints

- Retention of a drug within liposomes is dependent on the drug solubility/lipophilicity and the bilayer composition.
- Drugs can also be actively loaded and entrapped within liposomes using pH gradients to manipulate the drug solubility.
- Liposomes composed of lipids with longer acyl chains, combined with cholesterol, generally show enhanced drug retention.

Factors influencing drug loading and retention in liposomes

As already discussed, the association of a drug with delivery systems such as liposomes can significantly change the pharmacokinetics and biodistribution of the drug. When the drug is associated with the liposome it is biologically inactive, protected from degradation and has the same pharmacokinetic profile as the liposomes. Upon release the drug is then biologically active, but not protected from degradation and the pharmacokinetic profile is then dictated by the drug attributes. Therefore it is important to consider drug retention within liposome systems. Not all drugs are stably retained by liposomes and a particular characteristic to consider is the drug solubility/lipophilicity.

Three categories of drug types may be differentiated in terms of their incorporation and retention in liposomes:

- Hydrophilic drugs (log $P < 1.7$): these are retained well in the aqueous core of liposomes.
- Lipophilic drugs (log $P > 5$): these are easily incorporated and retained within the liposome bilayers.
- Intermediate drugs (log P 1.7–5): these partition between the bilayer and aqueous phase, which can result in rapid loss from the liposome.

As drugs with intermediate log P values can be difficult to deliver with liposomes due to their poor retention, alternative mechanisms to promote drug entrapment and retention within the liposomes have to be adopted.

Remote loading of doxorubicin into liposomes

If these drugs are weak acids or weak bases, the pH or chemical composition of the internal aqueous compartment of the liposomes can be manipulated so that the drug concentrates into complexes in the interior. This can result in high drug retention within the liposomes. This method has been described as active loading, remote loading or pH gradient loading and has been used for drugs including doxorubicin, daunorubicin and vincristine. These drug complexes can also help retain the drug within the liposomes.

Liposomes are prepared with ammonium sulphate entrapped within the aqueous phase. This is achieved by preparing liposomes in the appropriate concentration of ammonium sulphate and subsequently removing the ammonium from the external phase by 'washing' the liposomes by dialysis or via gel filtration. This results in an ammonium sulphate gradient across the liposome bilayer with high concentrations of sulphate within the liposome aqueous core, which acts as a counterion for amphipathic weak bases such as doxorubicin. To load the liposomes, doxorubicin HCl is added to the external media and the neutral form of the doxorubicin can diffuse across the liposome bilayer and enter the aqueous phase of the liposome. The doxorubicin then forms a drug–sulphate complex within the liposome, resulting in the formulation of a gel-like precipitate which becomes trapped within the liposomes (Figure 8.13). A similar method can be used for loading of amphipathic weak acids where cations such as calcium can be used to create the gradient. Using these methods, loading efficiencies of >90% can be achieved.

Durg retention within liposomes
The integrity of a liposome and its drug retention properties are also dramatically influenced by bilayer composition. The two main factors are:
1. Lipid structure: the acyl chain length and the degree of saturation of the lipids creating the bilayer both influence drug retention. As the acyl chain length of the phospholipid increases, the transition temperature of the phospholipid generally increases. This increase in acyl chain length is also known to correspond to an increase in drug retention, therefore longer acyl chain lipids can improve drug retention within liposomes. The presence of unsaturated bonds within the acyl chain (e.g.

Figure 8.13 Doxil drug loading by ammonium ion gradient method.

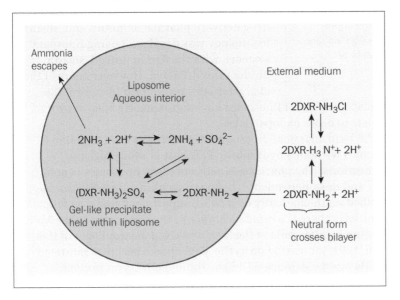

distearoylphosphatidylcholine) will reduce the transition temperature of the system and increase the bilayer permeability, thereby increasing drug leakage from the liposomes.

2. Cholesterol content: the presence of cholesterol is known to influence the release properties of liposomes. Increasing the cholesterol content of a liposome formulation up to a maximum of 50 mol% can improve drug retention within liposomes. This is thought to be due to the ability of cholesterol to reduce the mobility of the phospholipids within the bilayer and thereby reduce the permeability of the bilayer.

Liposomes for sustained release

DepoCyt (cytarabine liposome injection) contains the antimetabolite cytarabine, encapsulated into multivesicular (non-concentric multiple bilayer) liposomes. Cytarabine, the active ingredient, is encapsulated in liposomes composed of dioleoylphosphatidylcholine (DOPC), cholesterol, triolein and dipalmitoylphosphatidylglycerol (DPPG). The liposomes are used to give a sustained release of cytarabine, an antineoplastic agent, after direct injection into the cerebrospinal fluid. The formulation is indicated for the intrathecal treatment of lymphomatous meningitis and is supplied as a liquid suspension.

KeyPoints

- Liposomes without a hydrophilic 'stealth' coat are cleared rapidly by the MPS and their pharmacokinetics is dose-dependent.
- Size, charge, phase transition temperature, cholesterol content and dose all influence the clearance rates of liposomes.

Pharmacokinetics of liposomes – 'classic' versus 'stealth' formulations

Liposomes are now well established as parenteral drug delivery systems for a range of drugs (Table 8.3) and on this basis it is no surprise that the majority of the work supporting the development of particulate drug delivery pharmacokinetics and 'stealth' technology was developed using liposome systems, with the first approved 'stealth' product Doxil/Caelyx. However many of the characteristics recognised to control the pharmacokinetics of liposomes have subsequently been shown to translate to other nanoparticles.

The term 'classical' liposomes is sometimes used to define liposomes without a hydrophilic PEG coat or other surface modifications. The pharmacokinetics of these liposomes is non-linear and dose-dependent. This pharmacokinetic profile can be described mathematically by a two-compartment model as follows.

Initially there is a rapid clearance of the liposomes by the MPS, including Kupffer cells of the liver and fixed macrophages of the spleen. With increasing dose, the MPS uptake becomes saturated and this rapid clearance will have limited effects on plasma concentrations if high doses are given. A second slower phase of liposome elimination then follows. This has been suggested to reflect recycling of MPS binding sites and/or recruitment of new MPS cells. The overall pharmacokinetic profile of these non-stealth 'classic' liposomes is influenced by a range of parameters, including:

- Liposome size: liposome clearance increases with increased liposome size.
- Liposome charge: charged liposomes (positive or negative) are cleared more rapidly than neutral liposomes.
- Phase transition: liposomes prepared with high transition temperature lipids (longer saturated acyl chains) are cleared slower than liposomes prepared with low transition temperature lipids.
- Cholesterol content: this can reduce clearance of the liposomes, possibly by decreasing interactions with lipoproteins.
- Dose: increasing the dose can saturate MPS uptake and reduce clearance.

Sterically stabilised 'stealth' liposomes have been shown to have a log linear and dose-independent clearance profile over a wide dose range. As discussed in previous sections, the presence of the hydrophilic polymer coating can reduce MPS recognition and clearance to give longer circulation times and promote passive targeting via the EPR effect.

Classical liposome formulations versus stealth liposome formulations

There are three commercial liposome formulations of anthracyclines, all with very different formulations.

1. *Myocet*: these are liposomes of ~180 nm in size, entrapping doxorubicin. They are composed of egg phosphatidylcholine and cholesterol (55:45 mol %) so fit within the 'classical' liposomes category. Due to their size, the liposomes are rapidly taken up by the MPS. This avoids peak plasma levels and reduces toxicity. The liposomes cleared by the MPS are then thought to create an 'MPS depot' from which drug re-enters the blood stream, mimicking a slow infusion. As a result tissue concentrations are comparable to the same dose of doxorubicin HCl administered as solution. The recommended dosage is 60–75 mg/m^2 every 3 weeks.

2. *Caelyx/Doxil*: this contains doxorubicin entrapped within liposomes 80–100 nm

Tip

There remains some debate regarding the true mechanism of doxorubicin in stealth liposomes. Whilst it is clear that stealth liposomes modify the pharmacokinetics and reduce toxicity of their entrapped drugs, the mechanism behind the reduced clearance is less clear, with some studies suggesting clearance is dose-dependent in animal studies. Studies have also suggested the formulation impairs liver macrophage function, reducing their ability to clear the formulation. Accelerated blood clearance of PEGylated liposomes upon repeated injections has also been noted in animal studies and may be a result of antibodies generated against PEG.

in size. The liposomes are composed of hydrogenated phosphatidylcholine, cholesterol, PEG_{2000}-distearoyl phosphatidyl ethanolamine, α-tocopherol (56:38:5:0.2 mol %). The PEG_{2000}-coating gives the liposomes the 'stealth' properties and the α-tocopherol is used as an antioxidant in the formulation. This formulation is used for the treatment of solid tumours, including Kaposi sarcoma and ovarian cancer. It is supplied as a sterile, red liposomal dispersion and must be diluted in 250 mL of 5% dextrose prior to administration. Once diluted it should be refrigerated and administered within 24 hours. It has a terminal half-life of ~4 days and shows preferential accumulation in tumours due to the EPR effect. The recommended dosing is 20–50 mg/m^2 every 3 or 4 weeks depending on the indication. Multiple dosing is limited by palmar–plantar erthrodysaesthesia, which is also known as hand–foot syndrome, and is caused by drug accumulation in the skin of the palms and soles of the patient's feet causing skin ulceration, blisters or sores.

3. *DaunoXome*: these liposomes are composed of distearylphosphatidylcholine (DSPC):cholesterol (2:1 mol ratio) and have a diameter of 45 nm with entrapped daunorubicin. DaunoXome is indicated for the treatment of advanced human immunodeficiency virus (HIV)-related Kaposi's sarcoma. It is available in a single-use vial for intravenous infusion and the liposome dispersion should appear red and translucent. The liposome formulation helps to target the daunorubicin to solid tumours selectively. Whilst this is not a 'stealth' formulation, tumour targeting is still noted with this formulation presumably due to the high transition temperature lipids used (DSPC) and the small vesicle size which helps prolong blood residence time.

KeyPoint

- Liposomes can be designed to break down in low-pH environments and this can aid drug escape from the endosomal compartment after cellular uptake of liposomes.

Intracellular targeting of drugs using liposomes

Cells with phagocytic activity will take up liposomes into endosomes which have a pH of ~5. Lysosomes will then fuse with the endosomes to form secondary lysosomes, where the lysosomal enzymes will break down the liposomes and their drug payload (depending on its structural attributes). Therefore drug degradation in the lysosomes is a major problem if drug delivery into the cytoplasmic compartment of the cell is required. Liposomal membranes can be prepared to be pH-sensitive and in a low-pH environment the liposome can destabilise and break down. It is thought that the break down of these pH-sensitive liposomes in the endosome may in turn cause the endosomal membrane to break down and the encapsulated drug to be released. pH-sensitive liposomes normally contain dioleoyl phosphatidylethanolamine (DOPE), which is not able to form liposomes in its own right and requires additional lipids to form liposomes. Such liposome systems are also referred to as fusogenic liposomes. Various other mechanisms, including the conjugation of trans-activating transcriptional activator proteins from HIV to liposomes, have also been investigated in preclinical studies.

Liposomes as vaccine delivery systems

In addition to passively targeting tumour sites, liposomes can also be used to target cells of the immune system such as dendritic cells and thereby enhance the delivery of antigens. As shown in Table 8.3, liposome-based vaccine systems are commercially available. Liposomes and related vesicle systems are known to induce humoral and cellular immunity to a wide range of antigens and in particular are useful for the delivery of soluble antigens which have a good safety profile but are weak at inducing immune responses. Due to their particulate nature, liposomes can adsorb or entrap soluble antigens, giving them particulate properties and thereby enhancing their immunogenicity. The composition of liposomes is known to influence their adjuvant efficacy and the clinically available products are prepared with influenza viral envelope components (virosomes). The use of viral membrane components, such as influenza haemagglutinin, allows the vesicles to have the same fusogenic properties of the native virus without the risks associated with using live virus-based vaccines: the virosomes enter antigen-presenting cells in a similar way to natural infection by influenza viruses using haemagglutinin-mediated endocytosis followed by fusion of the virosomal and endosomal membrane, which results in antigen presentation.

> **KeyPoints**
>
> - Liposomes can also be used to target vaccines to cells of the immune system.
> - Virosomes can be prepared to incorporate influenza viral membrane components and used to enhance immune responses to antigens. These systems are used clinically.

Vesicle-based vaccines

- *Epaxal.* This is a hepatitis A vaccine containing inactivated hepatitis A virus. The inactivated virus has been adsorbed on to virosomes. Virosomes are small vesicle structures, ~150 nm in size, prepared from the outer coat of influenza virus and additional phospholipids. Epaxal is reported to induce protective antibodies within 10 days of vaccination and after the second booster injection it provides seroprotection for at least 20 years.
- *Inflexal V.* This is a virosomal influenza vaccine. Haemagglutinins, isolated from the influenza virus envelope,

are purified and combined with lipids to form virosomes. The influenza virus is subject to various mutations which result in different strains circulating. These strains have different antigenic profiles so the vaccine needs to be matched to the strain. Information on circulating strains is gathered by the World Health Organization and vaccine antigen composition is modified annually to follow the World Health Organization recommendations for each year.

Passive targeting of photodynamic therapy using liposomes
Visudyne (Table 8.3) is a light-sensitive delivery system that has been approved by the US Food and Drug Administration. It is a liposomal formulation used to treat age-related macular degeneration which can result in vision loss. The liposomes are composed of dimyristoyl phosphatidylcholine and egg phosphatidylglycerol that entrap the photosensitiser verteporfin. The liposomes are given by intravenous infusion, and they are selectively retained in the neovascular spots of the eye, which promotes passive targeting of the dye due to the enhanced permeability and slow clearance of colloidal systems from these areas. Thus the liposomes act as a delivery system to localise the photosensitising compound selectively to the target tissue. Fifteen minutes after the start of the injection the now localised liposome system is activated via a non-thermal laser light which promotes the liposomes to release their content by oxidative degradation of the lipid bilayer and the activation of the photosensitising agent (verteporfin). This promotes light-induced toxicity, reducing undesirable cell proliferation.

KeyPoints

- Microspheres are spherical particulates in the micrometre size range. They can give controlled release and also targeted delivery in some instances.
- They may also be beneficial as vaccine delivery systems.

Microspheres and microcapsules
As their name suggests, microspheres are spherical particles with diameters in the micrometre size range. Microspheres can be manufactured to be solid, porous or hollow, with the latter commonly being referred to as microcapsules. Their composition and preparation are basically the same as for nanoparticles, with both natural and synthetic polymers being used in their preparation. The polymers used in their preparation can be selected to control drug release based on the degradation rate of the polymers. As with nanoparticles, the most commonly used polymers are PLA and PLGA. Due to their larger size, microspheres are not suitable for intravenous injection but have been investigated for drug delivery through a variety of routes, including oral delivery, pulmonary delivery, ocular applications and nasal delivery. In many of these instances

microspheres are acting as a controlled-release system rather than a targeted system: for example, PLGA microparticles have been investigated as possible systems to give local controlled drug delivery to the brain similar to Gliadel (Chapter 6).

For pulmonary drug delivery and vaccine delivery these systems can also be described to enhance targeting of drugs. For drug delivery to the lung, microspheres can be tailored to have an optimum aerodynamic diameter that allows targeting to the various regions of the lung. For example, the use of microspheres to target drugs such as rifampicin to the alveolar macrophages within the lung has been investigated as a possible means of improving treatment of tuberculosis by decreasing doses and reducing the systemic side-effects that are commonly seen with oral tuberculosis treatments.

Microspheres as vaccine delivery systems

Similar to liposomes, microspheres are able to enhance the delivery of antigens to cells of the immune systems and enhance vaccine efficacy. The uptake of microspheres by phagocytic cells is well documented and this uptake into antigen-presenting cells is an important attribute of particulate vaccine adjuvants. The appropriate size for uptake of microspheres appears to be in the range of 1–3 μm and cationic systems appear to be particularly effective for uptake into macrophages and dendritic cells. In the development of vaccine delivery systems the selection of the route of administration is important and application of the delivery systems for mucosal administration can be improved by the use of absorption enhancers such as chitosan.

With these systems both antigen loading within the microspheres and antigen adsorption to the surface have been investigated. Several reports have noted that adsorption of the antigen to the surface of the microspheres produced similar or higher immune responses compared to antigen being entrapped within microspheres, with the additional advantage that adsorption to the surface of the particles avoids the exposure of antigen to organic solvents and high shear stresses during formulation and low pH conditions inside the microparticle caused by polymer degradation.

Tip

Microspheres can be prepared by similar processes to polymer nanoparticles using single-emulsion and double-emulsion procedures.

Tip

After inhalation particles < ~5 μm in diameter generally show efficient delivery into the lung. Particle sizes between 3 and 5 μm deposit predominantly in the terminal bronchiole region and particles below 3 μm have good deposition within the alveolar region.

Tip

Tuberculosis is a major global killer. The causative agent, *Mycobacterium tuberculosis,* enters the lung via inhalation and is then phagocytosed by alveolar macrophages, where it remains alive. It is difficult to achieve appropriate drug concentrations to these sites after oral therapy.

Summary

In this chapter we have seen that there are many options when considering drug carriers for site-specific drug targeting. The majority of these systems exploit passive targeting mechanisms using the natural attributes of the carrier in combination with the clearance mechanisms within the body, with antibodies being the main systems offering active targeting. However the combination of antibody targeting with drug carrier systems may offer the potential for further improvement in active targeting in clinical products.

Self-assessment

After having read this chapter you should be able to:

- describe the various options available for drug targeting
- discuss, with the use of examples, how prodrugs can be designed to give site-specific localisation and discuss the limitations of using prodrugs for drug targeting
- list the various types of carrier systems that can be used to promote drug targeting
- draw the structure of an IgG antibody, identifying the Fab and Fc regions, and the variable and constant regions
- discuss how polyclonal antibodies can be used for passive immunisation
- describe how botulism antitoxin can be used in the postexposure prophylaxis treatment of botulism
- describe the difference between monoclonal and polyclonal antibodies and explain how monoclonal antibodies are used therapeutically
- discuss how monoclonal antibody therapies actively target drugs
- discuss how Rimicade and Herceptin work
- compare the actions of Mabthera and Bexxar in their ability to cause targeted B-cell death
- describe the molecular design of a polymeric conjugate which can improve the targeting of chemotherapeutic drugs.
- discuss examples of polymer conjugates that are used clinically, identifying their polymer backbone, their conjugated drug and their mechanism of drug targeting
- compare and contrast dendrimer drug delivery systems to micelles, describe each system, discuss how they can be used to target drugs and their respective advantages and disadvantages
- discuss the advantages and disadvantages of macromolecular drug targeting
- describe how you would design a particulate system to avoid MPS uptake and rapid clearance by the liver
- explain why 'stealth' particulate systems target tumour sites

- discuss if 'stealth' coatings should be used in actively targeted nanoparticles
- discuss Abraxane. Is this an example of a passively or actively targeted delivery system?
- discuss the problems of using Cremophor EL as a means of delivering paclitaxel
- describe what liposomes are, and why they are able to incorporate hydrophilic and lipophilic drugs
- describe, compare and contrast the three lipid formulations of amphotericin B
- with reference to the critical packing parameter, discuss how the lipid geometrical shape influences how the lipids self-aggregate
- identify commonly employed lipids used in the formulation of liposomes
- describe how one should design a liposome formulation to give good stability and high drug retention
- in comparison to liposomes, identify two alternative vesicle-based delivery systems and discuss their potential applications
- compare the pharmacokinetics of 'classical' versus 'stealth' liposomes and discuss the mechanisms of drug delivery of Myocet compared with Caelyx
- explain what virosomes are and how they work as vaccines
- describe how microspheres can be designed to target the delivery of drugs against tuberculosis.

Questions

1. **Indicate which of the following statements is/are not correct (there may be more than one answer).**
a. Prodrugs can be defined as compounds which undergo biotransformation after exhibiting a biological response.
b. Prodrugs can be formulated to promote site-specific localisation.
c. L-dopa is an amino acid prodrug of carbidopa and is actively transported across the blood–brain barrier.
d. Carbidopa, a decarboxylase inhibitor, inhibits conversion of L-dopa in the circulation and peripheral tissue.
e. Carbidopa does not cross the blood–brain barrier.

2. **Indicate which of the following statements is/are not correct (there may be more than one answer).**
a. Soluble drug carriers generally have a greater ability to extravasate compared to particulate carriers.
b. Soluble macromolecular carriers, including antibodies, polymers and proteins, can be used to support site-directed drug targeting.

c. Soluble drug carriers can in general carry a larger drug load
    compared to particulate systems.
d. The covalent attachment of the drug to a soluble drug carrier
    may inhibit the activity of the drug.
e. As actively targeting systems, the plasma half-life of soluble drug
    carriers is independent of their molecular weight, ionic nature,
    configuration and interaction with biological components in
    circulation.

3. **Indicate which of the following statements is/are not correct
    (there may be more than one answer).**
a. Antibodies are large proteins produced by T cells.
b. Antibodies are also known as immunoglobulins.
c. Antibodies can target antigens and so can be used as targeted
    drugs in their own right.
d. Antibodies can be used as targeting groups which are conjugated
    to other drugs or carrier systems.
e. Whilst there are several classes of antibodies, most clinically
    approved products are based on immunoglobulin IgA antibodies.

4. **Indicate which of the following statements is/are not correct
    (there may be more than one answer).**
a. Monoclonal antibodies are produced from a single-cell
    hybridoma cell line.
b. Chimeric antibodies are composed of murine variable regions
    fused with human constant regions.
c. Humanised antibodies are produced by grafting murine
    hypervariable amino acid domains into human antibodies.
d. Adalimumab is a human antibody, used in the treatment of
    persistent, aggressive human epidermal growth factor receptor-2
    (HER2)-driven metastatic cancers.
e. Rituximab is a chimeric antibody, used in the treatment of
    follicular and non-Hodgkin's lymphoma.

5. **Indicate which of the following statements is/are not correct
    (there may be more than one answer).**
a. Antibodies can be used to target drugs and as targeting groups
    for other drug carriers.
b. Ibritumomab tuixetan (Zevalin) is a human anti-CD20 antibody
    conjugated to yttrium 90.
c. Tositumomab (Bexxar) is a murine anti-CD20 antibody
    conjugated to iodine 131.
d. The cytotoxin delivered by gemtuzumab (Mylotarg) is
    doxorubicin.
e. Gemtuzumab (Mylotarg) is a humanised anti-CD33 antibody–
    cytotoxin conjugate targeting leukaemia cells.

6. **Indicate which of the following statements is/are not correct (there may be more than one answer).**
a. Drugs can be conjugated to polymers to enhance the site-specific targeting via both passive (enhanced permeability and retention (EPR) effect) and active targeting mechnisms.
b. Overall these polymer–drug conjugate systems are generally larger than 200 nm in size.
c. There are generally three basic components to polymer–drug conjugate delivery systems: a water-soluble polymer, a linker and the drug.
d. Synthetic polymers such as hydroxypropylmethacrylate (HPMA) copolymers, poly(ethyleneglycol) (PEG) and poly(glutamic acid) (PGA) are the most commonly used polymeric soluble drug carriers.
e. PEG and HPMA are biodegradable polymers, whilst PGA is not.
f. Examples of linkers include amine, carbamate and ester groups.

7. **Indicate which of the following statements is/are not correct (there may be more than one answer).**
a. Particulate drug delivery systems are generally unaffected by cells of the mononuclear phagocyte system (MPS).
b. Particulate drug delivery systems include dendrimers, nanoparticles, micelles, liposomes and microspheres.
c. The ability of larger particles to leave the systemic circulation may be limited.
d. Using particulate drug delivery systems it is generally required to conjugate the drug to the delivery system covalently.
e. Drugs carried by particulate drug delivery systems may be protected from degradation during transit to the target site.

8. **Indicate which of the following statements is/are not correct (there may be more than one answer).**
a. PEGylation is the most frequently adopted method to impart a lipophilic coating on particulate drug delivery systems.
b. PEGylation masks the surface characteristics of the particulates, suppressing interactions of opsonins with the particle surface.
c. PEGylation of particles can only be achieved by chemically conjugating polymer chains on to the surface of the particle.
d. Clinically most particulate drug delivery systems available exploit passive targeting via the MPS or the EPR effect.

9. **Indicate which of the following statements is/are not correct (there may be more than one answer).**
a. Dendrimers are branched polymer macromolecules.
b. Dendrimers form spontaneously by the addition of suitable monomers.

c. Dendrimers can be designed for passive targeting with a PEG coat.

d. Dendrimers can be designed for active targeting without the need of the addition of targeting groups.

e. Drugs can either be covalently bound to the dendrimer structure or solubilised within hydrophobic regions of the structure.

10. Indicate which of the following statements is/are not correct (there may be more than one answer).

a. Solid polymeric nanoparticles are most commonly prepared from poly(lactide-co-glycolide) (PLGA), polylactic acid (PLA), polycaprolactone (PCL) and polysaccharides (particularly chitosan).

b. Polymeric nanoparticles are usually prepared by the lipid hydration method.

c. Solid lipid nanoparticles are colloidal particles made of solid lipids (e.g. solid triglycerides, saturated phospholipids and fatty acids) and are dispersed in an organic phase (usually hexane).

d. Typically solid lipid nanoparticles are produced by either hot or cold homogenisation.

e. Proteins can also be used for the construction of nanoparticles, and the first commercial product based on protein nanotechnology is Abraxane, containing the drug doxorubicin and used for the treatment of breast cancer.

11. Indicate which of the following statements is/are not correct (there may be more than one answer).

a. Block copolymers with amphiphilic properties (due to large solubility differences between their hydrophilic and hydrophobic groups) may be used for the delivery and targeting of drugs.

b. Compared to surfactant micelles, polymeric micelles are generally less stable and have higher critical micellar concentrations.

c. The hydrophobic part of polymeric micelles may also provide steric stabilisation and 'stealth' coating to the constructs.

d. The hydrophilic part of polymeric micelles often comprises polyaspartate, polylactide or polycaprolactone.

e. Immunomicelles may be prepared by the chemical attachment of monoclonal antibodies to reactive groups in the hydrophilic part of polymeric micelles.

12. Indicate which of the following statements is/are not correct (there may be more than one answer):

a. Liposomes are closed spherical vesicles consisting of an aqueous core surrounded by one or more concentrically arranged bilayer membranes.

b. There are no liposome products currently available for clinical use.
c. Liposomes are usually composed of natural or synthetic lipid molecules, with phospholipids being most often used.
d. Through modification of the bilayer composition the drug release rate of entrapped drugs can be controlled.
e. Liposomes as drug delivery systems can encapsulate hydrophilic drugs (within their bilayer regions) and solubilise lipophilic drugs (within the core of the liposome).

13. **Indicate which of the following statements is/are not correct (there may be more than one answer):**
a. The shape of the lipid may be expressed by its critical packing parameter (p).
b. The aggregation state of polar lipids is largely independent of changes in pH, temperature and lipid concentration.
c. Polar lipids with $p < 1/3$ generally form spherical micelles.
d. Polar lipids with p values between 1/3 and 1/2 generally form cylindrical micelles.
e. Polar lipids with $p > 1/2$ may form planar bilayers or inverted micelles.

14. **Indicate which of the following statements is/are not correct (there may be more than one answer):**
a. Liposomes disperse spontaneously as they are thermodynamically stable systems.
b. Phosphatidylcholine is a zwitter-ionic phospholipid.
c. Phosphatidylglycerol has a negatively charged head group.
d. The transition temperature of lipids is defined as the temperature above which the lipid physical state changes from the ordered gel phase to the disordered liquid crystalline phase.
e. The presence of cholesterol within liposome formulations improves stability of liposomes in vitro, but not in vivo.

15. **Indicate which of the following statements is/are not correct (there may be more than one answer).**
    In addition to classical phospholipid-based vesicles, a range of related systems has been developed for drug delivery and targeting. These systems include:
a. Endosomes.
b. Niosomes.
c. Bilosomes.
d. Polymerised liposomes.
e. Lysosomes.
f. Virosomes.

16. **Indicate which of the following statements is/are not correct (there may be more than one answer):**
a. Multilamellar vesicles are vesicles which consist of a large number of concentric bilayers, with sizes ranging from 100 nm to several micrometres.
b. Due to their multiple bilayers, multilamellar vesicles are suited to encapsulation of lipophilic substances.
c. Small unilamellar vesicles consist of a single bilayer enclosing an aqueous core and theoretically can be as small as 5 nm.
d. Large unilamellar vesicles are single bilayer liposomes generally over 1000 nm in size.
e. Small unilamellar vesicles have a large surface curvature and a high membrane tension.
f. Large unilamellar vesicles have a larger aqueous core than the small unilamellar vesicles and can entrap high amounts of hydrophilic drugs.

17. **Indicate which of the following statements is/are not correct (there may be more than one answer):**
a. Hydrophilic drugs ($\log P > 1.7$) are usually retained well in the aqueous core of liposomes.
b. Lipophilic drugs ($\log P < 5$) are usually incorporated and retained well within the liposome bilayers.
c. Intermediate drugs ($\log P\ 1.7 - 5$) partition between the bilayer and aqueous phase, which can result in rapid loss from the liposome.
d. For intermediate drugs that are weak acids or weak bases, the pH of the internal aqueous compartment of the liposomes can be manipulated so that the drug concentrates in the interior (active loading).
e. Active loading has been used for the liposomal encapsulation of several drugs, including doxorubicin, daunorubicin and vincristine.

18. **Indicate which of the following statements is/are not correct (there may be more than one answer):**
The overall pharmacokinetic profile of 'classic' liposomes is influenced by a range of parameters, including:
a. Liposome size: liposome clearance increases in direct proportion to increased liposome size.
b. Liposome charge: charged liposomes (positive or negative) are cleared slower than neutral liposomes.
c. Phase transition: liposomes prepared with high transition temperature lipids (longer saturated acyl chains) are cleared faster than liposomes prepared with low transition temperature lipids.

d. Cholesterol: presence of cholesterol in the vesicle bilayers can reduce clearance of the liposomes.

e. Dose: increasing the liposome dose can saturate MPS uptake and reduce clearance.

19. **Indicate which of the following statements is/are not correct (there may be more than one answer):**

a. Caelyx contains doxorubicin entrapped within liposomes 80–100 nm in size.

b. The liposomes in Caelyx are composed of hydrogenated phosphatidylcholine, cholesterol, PEG_{2000}-DSPC and α-tocopherol.

c. The α-tocopherol gives the liposomes the 'stealth' properties and the PEG_{2000} is used as an antioxidant in the formulation.

d. This formulation is used for the treatment of solid tumours, including Kaposi sarcoma and ovarian cancer.

e. Caelyx has a terminal half-life of ~4 days and shows active targeting.

20. **Indicate which of the following statements is/are not correct (there may be more than one answer):**

a. Liposomal membranes can be prepared to be pH-sensitive and in a low-pH environment the liposome can destabilise and break down.

b. The breakdown of these pH-sensitive liposomes in an endosome may cause the endosomal membrane to break down and the encapsulated drug to be released.

c. pH-sensitive liposomes often contain dioleoylphosphatidylethanolamine (DOPE).

d. pH-sensitive liposome systems are also referred to as immunogenic liposomes.

e. DOPE is able to form liposomes in its own right and does not need the addition of other polar lipids.

21. **Indicate which of the following statements is/are not correct (there may be more than one answer):**

a. Liposomes can be used to target cells of the immune system (such as dendritic cells) and thereby enhance the delivery of antigens.

b. Liposomes can adsorb or entrap soluble antigens.

c. Immunogenicity of antigens is often enhanced if they are incorporated in particulate systems.

d. Some clinically used vesicles are prepared with influenza viral envelope components (so-called bilosomes).

e. The use of viral membrane components, such as influenza haemagglutinin, can give the vesicles fusogenic properties.

22. **Indicate which of the following statements is/are not correct (there may be more than one answer):**
a.   The use of microspheres to target drugs such as rifampicin to alveolar macrophages has been investigated as a possible means of improving the treatment of tuberculosis.
b.   Particles >~5 μm in diameter generally show efficient delivery into the lung.
c.   Particles with sizes between 3 and 5 μm deposit predominantly in the terminal bronchiole region.
d.   Particles above 3 μm have good deposition within the alveolar region.

Further reading

Prodrugs
Majumdar A *et al*. Membrane transporter/receptor-targeted prodrug design: strategies for human and veterinary drug development. *Adv Drug Deliv Rev* 56: 2004; 1437–1452.

Antibodies
Daugherty AL, Mrsny RJ. Formulation and delivery issues for monoclonal antibody therapeutics. *Adv Drug Deliv Rev* 58: 2006; 686–706.
Drewe E, Powell RJ. Clinically useful monoclonal antibodies in treatment. *J Clin Pathol* 55: 2002; 81–85.
Hale G. Therapeutic antibodies – delivering the promise?. *Adv Drug Deliv Rev* 58: 2006; 633–639.

Polymer conjugates
Garnett MC. Targeted drug conjugates: principles and progress. *Adv Drug Deliv Rev* 53: 2001; 171–216.
Vicent MJ, Duncan R. Polymer conjugates: nanosized medicines for treating cancer. *TRENDS Biotechnol* 24: 2006; 39–47.

Dendrimers
Boyd BJ. Past and future evolution in colloidal drug delivery systems. *Expert Opin Drug Deliv* 5: 2008; 69–85.

Micelles
Matsumura Y. Poly(amino acid) micelle nanocarriers in preclinical and clinical studies. *Adv Drug Deliv Rev* 60: 2008; 899–914.

Nanoparticles
Faraji AH, Wipf P. Nanoparticles in cellular drug delivery. *Bioorg Med Chem* 17: 2009; 2950–2962.
Moghimi SM *et al*. Nanomedicine: current status and future prospects. *FASEB J* 19: 2005; 311–330.
Torchilin VP. Multifunctional nanocarriers. *Adv Drug Deliv Rev* 58: 2006; 1532–1555.

Wong J *et al.* Suspensions for intravenous (IV) injection: a review of
development, preclinical and clinical aspects. *Adv Drug Deliv Rev* 60: 2008;
939–954.

Protein nanoparticles
Hawkins MJ *et al.* Protein nanoparticles as drug carriers in clinical medicine.
Adv Drug Deliv Rev 60: 2007; 876–885.

Lipid nanoparticles
Joshi MD, Müller RH. Lipid nanoparticles for parenteral delivery of actives.
Eur J Pharm Biopharm 71: 2009; 161–172.

Microemulsions
Date AA, Nagarsenker MS. Parenteral microemulsions: an overview.
Int J Pharm 355: 2008; 19–30.

Liposomes
Janoff AS (1999) *Liposomes – Rational Design.* New York: Marcel Dekker.

Niosomes
Uchegbu IF (2000) *Synthetic Surfactant Vesicles: Niosomes and Other
Nonphospholipid Vesicular Systems.* Amsterdam: Harwood Academic
Publishers.

Microparticles
Moshfeghi AA, Peyman GA. Micro- and nanoparticles. *Adv Drug Deliv Rev* 57:
2005; 2047–2052.
O'Hagen DT *et al.* Microparticle-based technologies for vaccines. *Methods* 40:
2006; 10–19.

Answers to self-assessment

Chapter 1

1. d
2. b
3. e
4. b
5. b
6. d
7. c
8. a
9. e
10. c

Chapter 2

1. a, c, e
2. a, d, e
3. a, b, e
4. a, c, d
5. b, c, e
6. b, c, d
7. a, b, e
8. c, d
9. a, c, e
10. a, c, d
11. a, e
12. a, c, d, e
13. b, c, d
14. b, c
15. b, d

Chapter 3

1. True
2. False
3. False
4. True
5. False
6. True
7. False
8. True
9. False
10. True
11. False
12. False
13. False
14. True
15. False
16. True
17. True
18. True
19. False
20. True

Chapter 4

1. b, e
2. b, c
3. b
4. a, d
5. b, c, e
6. c
7. b, e

Chapter 5

1. c, d
2. a, c, d
3. b, c
4. a, c
5. b, c
6. a, d, e
7. a, d
8. b, d
9. a, c, d
10. a, c
11. b, d
12. a, c, d
13. a, c
14. a, e

Chapter 6

1. a, b, e
2. b, c
3. b, d, e
4. a, b, c
5. a, d
6. a, c
7. a, b, c
8. a, b, e
9. a, b, d

Chapter 7

1. c
2. e
3. c
4. b
5. d
6. e
7. a
8. c
9. a
10. e
11. b
12. d

Chapter 8

1. a, c
2. c, e
3. a, e
4. d
5. b, d
6. b, e
7. a, d
8. a, c
9. b, d
10. b, c, e
11. b, c, d

12. b, e	16. c, d	20. d, e
13. b	17. a, b	21. d
14. a, e	18. b, c	22. b, d
15. a, e	19. c, e	

Mind maps

Minds maps are a useful way to organise and categorise information and can enhance your creative problem-solving abilities. Using mind maps can help you piece together and structure information. They are also quick to review and help to make information easy to remember. The best mind maps are the ones you make yourself, so we encourage you to change or expand the example mind maps we have provided for each chapter.

Chapter 1. Controlling drug delivery.

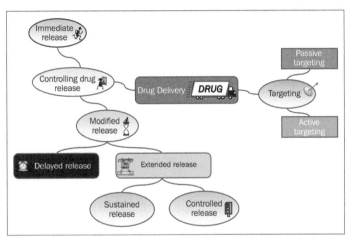

Chapter 2. Immediate-release drug delivery systems I: increasing the solubility and dissolution rate of drugs.

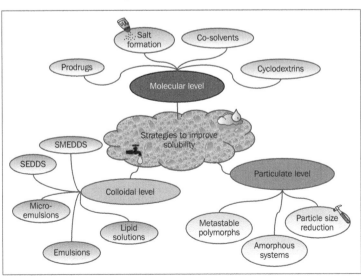

Chapter 3. Immediate-release drug delivery systems II: increasing the permeability and absorption of drugs.

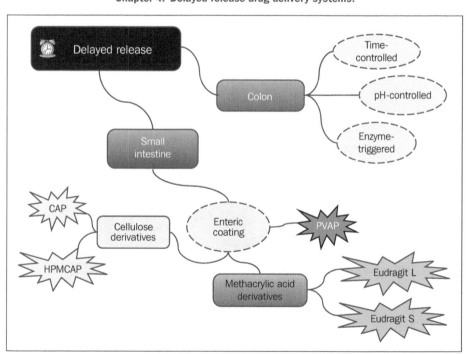

Chapter 4. Delayed-release drug delivery systems.

Chapter 5. Sustained-release drug delivery systems.

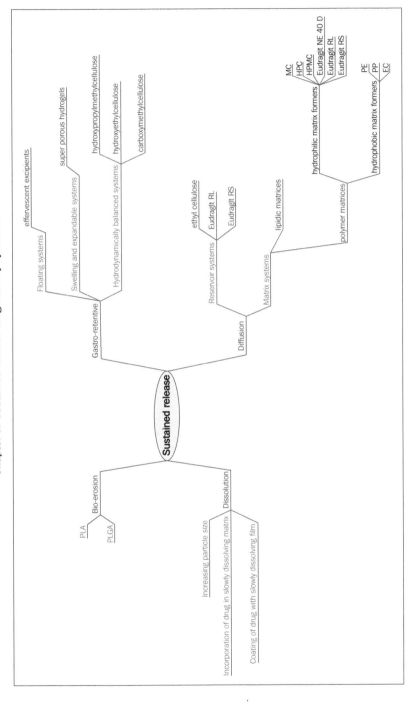

Chapter 6. Controlled-release dosage forms.

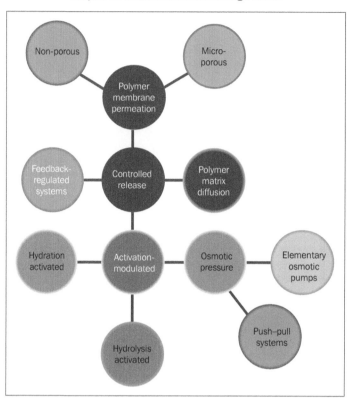

Chapter 7. Site-directed drug targeting.

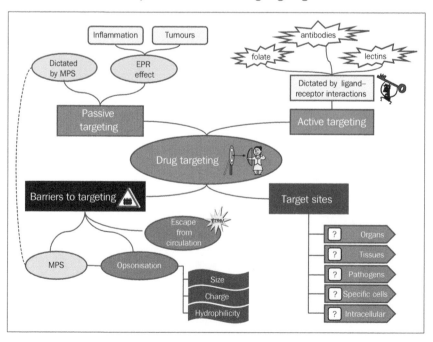

Chapter 8. Carriers for drug targeting.

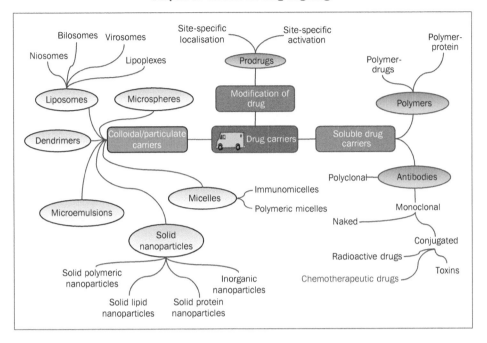

Index